TIGGY WALKER

BOTH SIDES NOW

Laughter, Grief and Everything in Between with Johnnie Walker

HarperCollins*Publishers*

HarperCollins*Publishers*
1 London Bridge Street
London SE1 9GF

www.harpercollins.co.uk

HarperCollins*Publishers*
Macken House, 39/40 Mayor Street Upper
Dublin 1, D01 C9W8, Ireland

First published by HarperCollins*Publishers* 2025
This paperback edition published 2026

1 3 5 7 9 10 8 6 4 2

A catalogue record of this book is
available from the British Library

ISBN 978-0-00-877006-8

Printed and bound in the UK using 100%
renewable electricity at CPI Group (UK) Ltd

To Johnnie,
with all my love.

'Darlin', I'll wait for you,
and should I fall behind,
wait for me'
Bruce Springsteen

FOREWORD

By Johnnie

Well, I guess you could say I've been a wild one all right. A typical Aries. When I met Tiggy I'd recently left rehab, so I was as clean as a whistle. It was a bit of a con, really, because you never lose that wild streak. It's part of your DNA, your energy, your drive. For years I called Tiggy 'a straight', which she was, not because she was dull – far from it; she lights up every room she enters – but because she was so sensible, with her feet firmly on the ground, unlike mine. I guess something in me recognised that stability in her and I thought, *I'll have some of that*. I need some of that. Of course, I really fancied her too. Her laugh, her energy, her blue eyes, her curves …

I've got a favourite record called 'The Joker' by Steve Miller Band, which includes the lines 'I really love your peaches/Wanna shake your tree'. And I did shake Tiggy's tree in more ways than one. I credit myself with opening her up to a more spiritual and less religious outlook on life. One of the first ideas I ever shared with her was that we are spirits on a human journey. I believe that we select the life we want to experience, getting a preview of all its joys and pitfalls before we make the final decision to take on the human form. Each human journey teaches us new lessons, until one day your soul has learned all it needs to from the human experience.

Tiggy chose a tough life, marrying me. Not only was I wild to her straight, which took some adjustment for us both, but I presented her with one health challenge after another. She's done far more caring of me than I would have wanted. She deserved so much more, and I genuinely wish I'd bought her more fun and less stress.

I've always admitted that apart from working hard on the radio, I can be pretty lazy. I act when I need to, but only then. Many is the time that I turned up five minutes before a show, giving my producers a high degree of stress, because I knew I could get away with it and I liked the energy from being on the edge. It's the same in my marriage. Tiggy is a producer and has the skills to run everything brilliantly. So, I've let her. As she says, I only work when there's a gun to my head or a mic in front of my mouth. Got to say, I've been bloody lucky – although I do think I've worn her out, which I feel bad about. She'll have a good rest when I'm gone.

I wish I'd earned more too. I would have loved to treat her to lavish holidays and amazing restaurants, both of which she would have adored. I've been terrible with money all my life, and it's thanks to her that we live in a house that we own and have had all the exciting trips we have. Just not on a luxury level. Not once has she ever been dissatisfied, though. As long as we were connected, she was happy.

I've been a radio man – one of a dying breed (literally) of jocks who went into this medium because we wanted to share the thing we were most passionate and excited about: music. It was never about fame or money. I know that Tiggy wouldn't have been attracted to me if it had been. She loves honest, real people. I know she's always respected me the most when she's watched me at work. I don't know why. A radio studio is just where I've always belonged, and so I guess working the desk and talking on mic became second nature to me. Over the years my music knowledge has earned me some brownie points too. She always reminded me how blessed I was to fall into the right job at such a young age. I was twenty-one. There is, however, a downside to being a radio man – which she also reminds me about. We're in the driving seat, often alone, with no one talking back to us. She is the opposite. A real people person who cares about those in her life. She's incredibly loved because she gives love. She's found it hard that I've lacked such qualities. Outspoken as she always has been with me, she said to me at our very final party at home, when I DJ'd live for the last time, 'Just because you're fucking dying doesn't mean you can be rude to everyone!'

I have been ill a lot and an introverted, insular DJ – with a wild streak. What did she do to deserve me? Well, as I tell her whenever she gets upset, 'Darlin' – you chose this life!'

I think we've learned a lot from each other. Marriage isn't easy, and somehow we've made it to the end, largely thanks to her forgiveness of my stupidities and failings. I do wonder where and when she and I will meet again. Will we live another life together, and if so, what will the relationship be? I pretty much know it will be her turn to lean on me. That is, if she ever needs to come back again.

I will end, as I always do, with a song, and if there's one I'd like to dedicate to her it would be Hal Ketchum's 'Loving You Makes Me a Better Man'. Because she has.

Loving you makes me a better man
These things I don't know how to do
You make me think I can

I've got a long way to go
But I know what I know like the back of my hand
Loving you makes me a better man

I've been wrong more than I cared to say
Time after time I've been lost
Just couldn't find my way

You shed a light on the path through the night
Leading right to the side where I stand
Loving you makes me a better man

I made mistakes, didn't have what it takes
Just to walk out, leave it alone
I've got a long lot of heartaches that follow me home

Time goes on, I watch it disappear
I've got a mind of my own
Now that I have you near

You came to me and it's easy to see
There's a line that I've crossed in the sand
Loving you makes me a better man
Loving you makes me a better man

Johnnie Walker, October 2024

THEN

LET THE MUSIC BEGIN

Ours is a love story. But it's so much more than that. It's a story of mistakes, challenges, changes, caring and an occasional sprinkling of stardust.

I had no inkling that you were to be a part of my life. I used to listen to you on Tuesday lunchtimes at Alton Convent doing the Radio 1 Chart Show when I was thirteen and you were twenty-nine. But after that I lost all knowledge of you. When Gordon, my songwriter 'Summer of 2001' fling, asked if I wanted to meet you, I was surprised. I thought you must be dead, having not heard your name in twenty-seven years. I declined the offer.

Monday nights were my sacrosanct yoga nights in Primrose Hill, but who was it who called me that evening so that it was too late for me to go? I've no idea. What I do know is, that call changed everything. Resigned to an evening at home, I made my sitting room a candlelit haven to do my own practice. I was deep into my asanas when the phone went again. It was Gordon. He'd already met up with you, yet you wanted to meet me too – because secretly you'd had a psychic inkling that I'd be important to you. It all seemed rather tiresome to have to shower, reapply make-up, get dressed and go back to Soho for the second time that day. I told Gordon I would meet you at The Union, my club in Greek Street. I wasn't fast getting there. I knew this was just Gordon's way of showing off that he had a girlfriend fifteen years younger than him. Men … I couldn't see him anywhere in the club. I was about to leave when suddenly before me there was Gordon, sat back on a sofa, grinning, and you were walking towards me with your hands outstretched. What an extraordinary sensation. I knew you. I recognised you. Not your face, but your being. Your soul, in fact. Here you were, my oldest friend who I had not seen for so long. And certainly not in this life. You kissed my cheek, sat me down next to you and we talked as if we were carrying on our conversation from our last life together. The connection was instant and total. It felt that there was so much we didn't need to say. So much we agreed on. And Gordon did not.

It cannot be denied that the timing of our meeting was strange. On a personal level and a global one. That day you had ended a long-running on/off relationship with your then girlfriend. Even though it had been a mutual decision, you were still in shock. To meet me on the same day did not allow you much recovery time – a fact that would bite us both very firmly on our backsides before long. The global situation almost felt pre-empted by us. We spoke of how spiritually bereft people in the West are. How materialistic. 'Something big has to happen to make people reassess their lives,' I suggested. The next day two planes flew into the Twin Towers.

I knew I would see you again. So did Gordon. Within ten days he ended it. While he never mentioned your name as the reason, I knew he was making space for you. He recognised that he was a stepping stone in my life. In other words, he wasn't going to get in our way. His reward for being so sensitive was being played on your Radio 2 *Drivetime* radio show, the song making the Radio 2 playlist, him getting a record deal and earning proper money for the first time in decades. He was very nearly the Christmas Number One. 'How Wonderful You Are' is a song I listen to with fondness, remembering the late, idiosyncratic, beautifully bonkers Gordon Haskell.

For you and me, a future lay ahead we could never have imagined.

I guess nothing about us as a couple was that normal. For a start, our deeper contact began when I sent a message to your Radio 2 *Drivetime* show about 9/11 – two days after we had met. I forwarded a fascinating email from an artist friend in Chicago with her reaction at the USA being attacked. While I didn't know what your show covered as I had never listened to Radio 2, I thought it might be interesting. But mainly it was a great excuse to contact you. I included my mobile number. On Friday afternoon I was in Dorset, where I owned a gorgeous cottage in the village of Ashmore. This was my weekend decompression place away from the bustle of Soho. I had grown up a country girl in

Hampshire, but at the age of sixteen announced that my future life would be in Dorset, following a one-day trip to Brownsea Island, compounded by a love of Thomas Hardy. As soon as I could afford to, I bought a property there. I was shopping in the local town of Shaftesbury when you called asking me out to dinner in London that night. I explained that I couldn't. You asked what I was up to. I blushed as I told you that I was just going into the florist as I was doing the church flowers that weekend. I had never done them before and indeed haven't since, but St Nicholas's Church in Ashmore had become a part of my life. I felt great comfort in the services each Sunday. In a village the church is also about community, and I was gently becoming part of Ashmore's, albeit on a weekend-only basis. I could hear the shock in your voice. Church flowers? Who is this woman? I felt so very un-rock 'n' roll and thought I'd probably blown it. Desperately back-peddling, I spluttered out that my sister Fiona was coming for the weekend to help me, because I couldn't do a flower arrangement to save my life. Happily, the utterly upper-middle-class-establishment image I'd managed to paint of myself in those two words, 'church flowers', did not put you off and we spent the weekend texting each other. Our first date was on the Monday evening – just one week after we met. It was a yoga class: my sacrosanct Monday night. You had told me when we met that you also did yoga. (Men!) So, taking you at your word, I booked us both into my regular class. You were already waiting for me in the light, airy reception area in

Primrose Hill when I arrived. You took my breath away. You were dressed head to toe in white, looking like a yoga guru. It was the first time I realised how attractive you were. It wasn't long into the class, as I looked back at you between my legs in Downward Dog, that I saw you were in total confusion. Limbs everywhere. I realised you had *never* done yoga. I cursed myself for messing up our first date. I'd made you look an idiot. Yet again, I thought I'd blown it. At the end of the longest ninety minutes, I rushed back to you and said, 'I'm so sorry, Johnnie.'

'What do you mean?' you said. 'I had all that time to admire your arse.'

After a quick supper at Manna vegetarian restaurant, when, to your annoyance, Simon the yoga teacher joined us, you drove me home in your old Saab. Before you set off you picked up a CD and put on a song: John Prine's 'All the Way With You'. I wondered if this was just a track you especially liked or if you were trying to tell me something. And if you were, was that something that you wanted to have sex with me, or spend your life with me? The latter seemed too far-fetched to contemplate. You stopped several times more on the short trip to Marylebone, putting on other songs. Were all your journeys so musically punctuated?

I asked you in for coffee (since you didn't drink in those days, still glowing in the goodness of rehab). You hated my flat. It was so neat, so Heal's, like a hotel. But as I tried to explain, my home and heart were in Dorset. We sat on opposite ends of the taupe suede sofa, longing to hold each other. We agreed that a hug was permissible and wouldn't be disloyal to Gordon, but the attraction was too great.

Our first kiss happened an hour later as you were about to leave. You leaned down to wish me goodnight and our lips met. If there was one moment in my life I could relive, it would be that. It felt as if we floated, and that a beautiful throng of angels flew silently around us, lifting us towards heaven. It was an out-of-body, out-of-this-world experience. We both felt it. Afterwards we looked into each other's eyes with a sense of wonder.

'Did I dream that we kissed last night?' I texted you in the morning.

'We did. And it was dreamy,' you assured me. I believe that what we experienced was pure love, and at that moment our two souls entwined and made a vow that whatever should come to pass, they would keep us together. And what two brave souls we have, for it seems that we were to be given one test after another, but they would not let us go. Even though at times I tried.

Next morning at Blink, the commercials production company where I was a producer, as everyone shared what they had done the night before, I casually mentioned I'd had a date with Johnnie Walker. There was a flurry of excitement from the production managers. James, the boss – a huge music fan – stayed silent at his desk, but seconds later Bachman–Turner Overdrive blasted out from his laptop: 'B-b-b-b-baby, you just ain't seen nothin' yet!' Everyone dissolved in laughter, including me.

I loved working at Blink. It was the best production company for commercials in Soho. I felt it was my reward after years in the business. Ten years before, I had opened my own production company, Wowhaus, in London, making commercials for Germany. I'd spent a year working at a production company in Munich, where I'd produced the commercials for visiting English and American directors, but generally, they were not that happy working in Germany – so I represented them for Germany, but based in London, where they could continue to use their familiar crews. The exchange rate was in our favour, it was a new concept and a great idea, except that potential clients were nervous of going with a new company in another country. We were a risk. After a year of selling hard in Frankfurt, Hamburg, Munich and Düsseldorf advertising agencies, renting out my flat to sofa surf and living on air, I felt the idea had failed. 'How many weeks can you hold on before the bank shuts you down?' asked my accountant, GT. The answer was three. 'Hold on!' he insisted. I did – and in came a Grundig TV commercial, and after that I never looked back. I sold the company after seven years, and when Blink asked me to join them I felt I had arrived at my natural home.

My first visit to your flat was a shock. At the opposite end of Marylebone High Street to mine, you rented a tiny, two-bedroom scruffy flat above Giraffe restaurant. Advertising was a world where we portrayed style, perfection and neatness. In my naivety I assumed that's how a successful BBC presenter would live. Far from it. Your furniture looked to be out of a charity shop. The flat was cramped, the bathroom grim, the kitchen in need of ripping out – everywhere was grubby because each surface was covered with stuff, and worst of all, thousands of CDs created chimney-like piles on every available bit of floor space. These weren't CDs you loved. These were ones you had been sent by the music pluggers who wanted nothing more than for Johnnie Walker to feature them on his show. Your reputation as a music influencer was still intact from your early pirate radio and Radio 1 days, when you had discovered many an act or artist. The strange thing for me was that, seeing all this music begging to be heard, my interest in new music got immediately crushed. Just by visiting your flat. Rather than a new CD being something exciting that I deliberately sought out, suddenly CDs represented pressure and untidiness. It was just too overwhelming to see them all begging to be heard. How could you differentiate between which ones would be good and which not? It was like huge amounts of homework. And honestly, you listened to so few of them. How could you do otherwise? There were so many. (Of course, as the years passed and everything became digital, that issue evaporated. Maybe you were sent masses of download links instead, which you could ignore. I didn't see them. Ironically, today, I still want to buy CDs rather than relying on streaming services. I prefer the physical to the digital.)

Your flat and mine: already it was clear we were very different people, and yet we continued to fall head over heels in love. Especially when you made it down to my Dorset cottage – the Clock House in Ashmore. I'm not sure you'd ever done country living. An AGA, a scrubbed white-painted table, an open fire, a well-stocked wine rack – it was all too much temptation, and after you had a mind coach called Tony Buzan as a guest on your *Drivetime* show, who told you that you were not alcoholic, you took the bold decision to share a bottle of red with me in front of the roaring fire. As it happens, Tony was right. While you would always prove yourself to have addictive traits, you were not an alcoholic, and I will always be grateful to Mr Buzan for telling you that. Sharing delicious bottles of red and white Burgundy has been one of our joys, and let's face it, we were both a bit freer when we'd had a glass or four.

My bedroom at the cottage had windows on two sides. You credit that and my Simon Horn sleigh bed with its amazing mattress as the reason for the best night's sleep you've ever had. I was so happy that you felt content there – until I went off riding my horse, Wicked Willy, when you did get a bit fractious and bored. No shop. No pub. Nothing. Ashmore has a dew pond, a church, a village hall, great walks and not a lot else. Not very rock 'n' roll.

There was much to learn about you. The radio stations, the two previous marriages, your two children, Sam and Beth (both in their twenties), your recent time in rehab and the reason you went there. The story that you were most ashamed about: that you had been sucked in by the 'fake sheikh' from the *News of the World*. He had met you to discuss a supposed radio show for somewhere in the Middle East. During this pretend negotiation he had said how hard it was to find good cocaine in London, and after much persuasion convinced you to chop out two lines of the white powder. You snorted yours but he declined his – which was when you smelled a rat. The hidden camera that took your photo meant you were on the front of the Sunday 'red top' paper. You had been 'stung'. (This front-page news is one thing you never showed me.) You were fired from Radio 2, went to rehab and had to fight in court to clear your name from the accusations as best you could. It would have been the end of your career had your ardent fans not saved you. The effects on you were enormous, not least financially, as you were left with enormous legal debts. Crikey – you certainly weren't the average date. Getting to know you was a mixture of heady excitement and deep alarm. One thing I could see early on: you were never going to be boring.

It wasn't long into our dating that you told me you would take me away for a weekend on your Harley-Davidson Fat Boy. Me on a motorbike – whatever next? Along with your biker friend Snapper we set off to Tintagel from my cottage. 'You're going to freeze,' you told me as I appeared in jeans and a Barbour jacket. You were right. It was a godforsaken challenge – uncomfortable, cold, mind-numbingly dull and lonely. We rocked up at the worst hotel I've ever seen. 'Isn't this fantastic?' you exclaimed. It reminded me of the first meal you took me to: a Thai in a scruffy café at the end of the King's Road, which during the day was an egg, chips and tea venue. A far cry from The Union, the Ivy and Quaglino's where I hung out in those days. Oh, Johnnie – how different our reference points were back then. The one notable moment of that trip was on a rock together on a north-Cornish beach. You asked me what my dreams were. 'To make a film called *ANTONIA* …' I said, and I told you the story of how my father had given me a beaten-up red book called *Antonia* by Naomi Jacob when I was sixteen. I was just departing for Umbria to stay with a distant family friend. It was my first solo trip and my first time to Italy. He told me to read it there because it was about an amazing Italian woman. He then added that it would make a great film. Deep within me, he had sown a seed, and the very first tender shoots were now eager to appear.

I returned the question and your reply was simply, 'To spend the rest of my life with you.' And coming home on a dark Sunday night, at a brightly lit petrol station where I bought a life-saving fleece, you looked into my eyes and I just knew you were nanoseconds away from proposing. Even then I knew you so well. But I think you also knew me, and that a service station under cruel strip lighting would not be the right setting for the story I would want to tell for the rest of my life.

Gigs after your *Drivetime* show soon became a part of our life: Ryan Adams, REM, Bruce Springsteen, Billy Joel, David Bowie, Brian Wilson, Elton John, Fleetwood Mac, Simon & Garfunkel, the Dixie Chicks, The Who, Neil

Diamond, The Rolling Stones, Eagles, Carly Simon, Crosby, Stills & Nash, mavericks like John Otway and many more, at London venues that ranged from Wembley Stadium, the Royal Albert Hall and the O2 to the smaller scale La Scala and Bush Hall. Our first gig together was James Taylor at the Hammersmith Apollo. I'd never listened to him before, which is extraordinary as he writes exactly the sort of music I enjoy – mellow and meaningful. It was my first experience of going backstage afterwards. How normal it all was. The large, badly lit room was quite un-special. James was relaxed and warm, greeting you like a cherished friend.

As we left and walked back to your car a punter shouted, 'Hi, Johnnie. Is that Sally Traffic with you?' and for the first time I revealed to you a spark of my fire as I responded to said punter:

'No, I'm bloody well not. I'm a lot younger than her.' How you laughed. Sally was your on-air bounce whom you had brought into the station to do the traffic news. You had great broadcast chemistry, but it was at times a feisty-sounding relationship.

I loved the Ryan Adams concert. I had never heard of him until I met you, and his album *Gold* was quickly one of my favourites. Watching him sing 'La Cienega Just Smiled', with you holding me from behind … It was bliss. And I must admit to some vanity. Many in the audience knew who you were. You were such a respected music man, and being the woman held by you made me feel a few inches taller – which at my height is a fabulous feeling.

A new motorbike made its entrance into your life: a BMW Road King. You announced that it was to be called Earl. You would be the Duke of Earl. At which we started singing, 'Duke, Duke, Duke, Duke of Earl, Earl, Earl …' You looked at me and said that made me your duchess. Thus, from the very early days of being together I called you Duke, and you called me Duchess, or usually Duch. Being someone with a recognisable voice, this proved to be very handy in public, as it must have reduced the JW sightings considerably as I never called you by your name.

The euphoria we experienced together in those first months was like nothing I have ever felt for its intensity and joy. We were nuts for each other. We were literally high on love.

When at the start of December I had to fly to Australia to shoot a Volvo car commercial, you rushed into the reception at Blink thirty minutes before you were due on air for the *Drivetime* show. 'What are you doing here? You should be at the studio!' I panicked.

You, cool as ever about time, handed me a package. 'Open it on the plane.' I did, some five hours later as the jumbo taxied along the runway. Inside was a MiniDisc player with a disc for me to listen to. And a Wright & Teague silver ring with the words 'Dedicated to the one I love'. It was the first song on your playlist. I cried so much that the air hostess came to check I was OK. It hurt me so much to be taking off and flying away from the man I loved so deeply.

We were only a few months into our relationship, but already you were dominating my every waking moment. You filled my heart. You were my reason to be. So when on the first day of filming the Volvo car ad in a New South Wales rainforest I got a text from your biker friend Snapper warning me that your ex was getting her claws back in, the earth crumbled beneath me. My director, Laszlo, was asking me what on earth had happened. My entire demeanour had changed, and the biggest day of car photography of my life was a total blur. I had no idea what awaited me on my return to England. But I knew it wasn't going to be good, and I dreaded it.

I landed back in England on Christmas Eve. As I pushed my trolley through the arrivals hall at Heathrow, looking for a driver holding a sign with my name on it, I noticed instead that the waiting crowd were enjoying a gorilla playing a guitar. All I could muster was a brief smile. Behind the gorilla stood a pantomime cow. Some reunion, I thought. It was only when I realised the gorilla was singing Gordon's new single 'How Wonderful You Are' that I turned around for a double-take. In a blur, the gorilla started laughing and the cow took its head off. Suddenly I was in your arms. You were laughing nervously. I was in shock.

A few hours later you, me, Gordon, Snapper (the unsung back of the cow) were in my kitchen in Dorset. Gordon – still our friend despite our break-up – always smoked, but suddenly for the first time ever I saw you light up a cigarette. But you had quit in rehab on Antigua – that relatively recent chapter of your life after the *News of the World* sting – what were you doing? I HATE smoking on a deep, pathological level. I could see you were on edge. I couldn't wait for the others to go. We needed to talk.

I was sitting on my white-painted kitchen table with you on the bench in front of me. I looked down into your eyes. 'What's been going on, Johnnie?' With alarming honesty, you confessed to visiting your recent ex and her child – who was not yours but to whom you had become an unofficial godfather (psychologically explained by you trying to make up for the lack of time you spent with your own daughter, Beth, when she was a young child) – and that she had done a big seduction number on you – candles, see-through negligee and cheap perfume. You tried to push her off, but that dark side of yours that finds temptation just too exciting ultimately could not resist. I know you didn't do the whole deed, but in my heart I felt you had betrayed me.

The bubble of our heady love had burst. I couldn't believe I could be stabbed so deep by an external act. It was two days before my forty-first birthday. I never had a period again. Years later, a consultant gynaecologist would tell me that shock can start the menopause. That act, that weakness of yours, that desperation of hers, I believe stopped us from ever having a child, and for you it was the start of an emotionally traumatic time that you always claimed was the cause of your cancer, which ultimately changed your health forever. You referred back to your regret of that slip for the next twenty years.

It wasn't the easiest Christmas. It was my first experience of your actions breaking a bit of me – just over three months after getting together. Defensively, you criticised me for living in the perfect world of advertising, of not knowing what hardship meant, of being a 'straight' (Me? A straight? I was far from that in my friends' eyes, always being a bit of a fun-loving party girl.) I fought back, telling you I had to sofa surf for a year when I started my own production company, working like crazy to get it going. You didn't want to hear that.

You got into such a state of feeling utterly guilty, confused and pulled between two women (for the record, I NEVER pulled – it's not the way I behave) that you ended everything, and for a few weeks I licked my wounds and built a protective zone around me. I loved my Dorset life. My horse, my cottage, my antidote to making commercials in the week. I never expected to hear from you again, but then on a Saturday evening in late January, when I was in my candle-lit bedroom meditating, you called. You were on Win Green – a mile away. You asked to come round, and in many ways that was my *Sliding Doors* moment. If I had told you to get lost and leave me alone, I would have gone on with my career and my stable, successful life. I would have been in control of my destiny and avoided a whole load of pain. But as it was, I felt sorry for you because it was cold and dark, and your voice – well, let's face it, you know how to use that voice. Around you came. As I have always said, you were my destiny – whether I wanted it or not.

In the three weeks of your absence I had done two things. I had told Blink I needed to leave and take a sabbatical. I was honestly so thrown by the emotion of the previous few months that I knew I wasn't performing as well as I should. My second act was thanks to my dear granny, who had left me £5,000 in her will. I decided to spend it on a month's Italian course in Florence, going out at the end of March. My E.M. Forster tribute trip to nurse my broken heart was starting on your fifty-seventh birthday. You asked if you could come out for that weekend. I was too weak to say no and start my adventure alone, even though it was supposed to be my time to heal. For those two nights I booked a hotel on the River Arno that I'd always fancied, the Hotel Lungarno.

It was here we experienced our first bit of magic together. An Italian plugger in the music business arranged for us to have an upgrade to the biggest suite. It was a huge room overlooking the Arno, with the crispest white sheets, white sofas, a bottle of bubbly on ice and white flowers on the enormous coffee table. It was as perfect as an advertising set. The next day a chauffeur arrived to drive us around Tuscany. He took us to medieval villages and Siena – one of my favourite Italian towns. I couldn't believe it. What a start to my month.

On Sunday we were free to walk the wonderful streets of Florence. Is it the olive skin of the men, or their beautiful dark hair? Whatever it was, the male inhabitants of the city unnerved you. At a bar on one side of the famous Ponte Vecchio you ordered a brandy, which you knocked back in one gulp. We walked to the centre of the bridge and watched the brown water flow slowly beneath us. You picked something off the ground and faced me. 'Tiggy, would you do me the greatest honour of becoming my wife?' I was stunned. 'Are you sure, Johnnie?' I kept repeating it. 'Are you sure?' I already had the measure of you. You had proved yourself to be an emotional, hot-headed decision maker, and also a touch possessive. It was fairly obvious that you did not want a Florentine man taking me away from you, so you were literally ring-fencing me for my four-week sojourn. You insisted you were sure, and put a Coca-Cola ring pull on my wedding finger.

At the hotel we drank the champagne. When you left early the next morning I was in a heightened state. You had convinced me that your intentions were true. We were getting married. And you wanted to do it in July. It was unbelievable. Only a couple of months before this you had ended it all. It seemed too amazing to be true, but of course I *wanted* it to be true, so I let it overtake my being. In my Italian conversation practice for the next four weeks, I could talk about only one thing: *mi sposo*.

While in Florence I went to Salvatore Ferragamo and bought the most expensive outfit I've ever purchased. Wide-legged trousers and a flouncy top in lilac, along with a pair of subtle-pink, high-heeled suede sandals. It was altered to fit me perfectly. This was my wedding outfit for July.

On my return home, speaking Italian a little better but still very much lacking, we went to the Larmer Tree Gardens

– home of the now-defunct Larmer Tree Festival – to talk about the wedding. We had missed meeting each other there by minutes when I was going out with Gordon. You saw he was one of the acts at the festival and had a Tannoy announcement put out for him, but we had left just five minutes before. Both of us love those gardens, which is why we chose them for our wedding venue. As a huge favour to us they squeezed an extra day into their schedule when they were due to be closed. We were shown where the ceremony could take place. There's a little round temple on the main lawn where we could do the honours. I was only joking when I called it the Temple of Doom, but as it happens that joke backfired on me.

Five weeks before the ceremony I collected the invitations from the printer, which were a postcard of the 'Temple of Doom' with the date on the back. I spent the weekend addressing the invitation envelopes. Alone. You had gone to visit your 'godchild' and ex for the weekend. This was something you had done about once a month, and while it made me feel uneasy, I would never have stopped you as you felt an emotional obligation towards the child. This particular weekend you didn't contact me once. Not even a text. By Monday my nerves were on edge. *Here we go*, I thought, *the next blow*. While I didn't need to call you to know what you were thinking, because already we were telepathically connected, I did just to be certain. I was right. You wanted to cancel the wedding. A right hook to my solar plexus. But it wasn't just the massive blow to my gut and heart. I had friends and family flying in from Australia, Italy and Germany, all so happy that I'd found the man of my dreams. I had to tell them, and everyone who had saved the date, that it was off. Oh, the humiliation. The indignity. The heartache. Made all the worse by the fact that you were bloody famous. I wrote a lame poem that you 'weren't quite ready to get wed at the end of July'. I was so brave. You didn't have to do a thing. You just went back to London to broadcast your *Drivetime* show. I couldn't listen that evening. The Salvatore Ferragamo outfit was put away, never to be worn. I've never spent so much on an outfit since.

Looking back at how accommodating and accepting I was that day, I believe I can only attribute it to our entwined souls. The belief, the knowing, that you were my destiny whether I wanted it or not. No matter how hard it would be. I could see your dilemma and suffering. The ex played on your incredibly susceptible guilt strings – something she knew how to do. And it was something that would be your Achilles' heel for several years to come. I'm proud that over our time together you would shed that coat of guilt, learning to believe in your inherent goodness rather than your weakness. That said, the scar of that day never completely healed in me. And the regret of it stayed with you to your grave.

You asked what I would do about the honeymoon that I'd booked at La Residencia in Deià, Mallorca. I told you that I was still going but would leave two days earlier so I wasn't around for what would have been the wedding day. You said you wanted to come too, since apparently the relationship wasn't over, just the ceremony. God, you had some gall. But oh, the immense amusement that I felt when we arrived and they said, 'Welcome Mr and Mrs Gatfield. Congratulations!' The hotel hadn't got the memo. And as I had booked it, they used my then surname – that of my previous husband, which I still used. Something competitive in me felt that you didn't hold all the cards after all. It was like a sharp slap for your poor behaviour. The bed was covered in red rose petals and a bottle of champagne on ice awaited us. We never opened it out of shame. I swept the petals away. I also slipped the silver ring 'Dedicated to the one I love' I was wearing on my wedding finger.

You always said that it was on our 'not the honeymoon' that you really fell in love with me. My instinct on the Ponte Vecchio had been utterly correct. But seeing how I behaved may have taught you something that you hadn't seen in me before, or indeed in any woman that you'd dated. Strength. Principles. Independence. You allowed yourself to let go, and one night as we sat naked together under a star-encrusted sky, making love in a jacuzzi, something in you connected – to me. You had never stayed anywhere quite so beautiful and luxurious. It made you feel better about yourself. Yes, you were worth this. You allowed your true self to be seen. You weren't the man ashamed of his *News of the World* drug sting, the man who had felt such paranoia and guilt. You were a man staying at one of the world's most gorgeous hotels with a woman you had fallen for but were afraid to commit to. You began to recognise that you and I were equals, destined to help each other. Both our souls were longing for you to realise that. We had an amazing nine days. On returning, you were determined to right the huge wrong and marry me. You compared us to Native Americans – a culture you always loved. You told me that they honeymoon before the wedding. If they return together the ceremony occurs; if apart, nothing happens and nothing is said. We returned together.

Our actual ceremony – to which we invited almost no one, as I was understandably petrified of another last-minute cancellation – took place in St Nicholas's Church, Ashmore, on Saturday, 21 December 2002. The Bishop of Salisbury had given us (both divorcees) dispensation to marry in church. In retrospect it was definitely worth waiting. We needed all of God's help to get us through the years ahead. As part of the ceremony you asked our friend Paul Venables to read out a piece you had chosen – 'The Invitation' by Oriah Mountain Dreamer. 'It doesn't interest me who you know – I want to know if you will stand in the centre of the fire with me and not shrink back …' Soon followed by 'Come on Baby Light My Fire' by The Doors as we walked down the aisle (played on the organ!).

A wedding lunch for my parents, all of our siblings, your dear son Sam, who was your best man, and our very closest friends (including Gordon) was held at the Museum Inn in Farnham, Dorset. Then we took a blustery drive down to the Dorset coast to the Anchor Inn at Seatown, as you wanted to wake by the sea. On the way there you received a text from your ex on news of the wedding: 'May God forgive you.' It was like a curse.

OUR TOP TEN MEANINGFUL SONGS

John Prine
ALL THE WAY WITH YOU
The first song you played me.

Hal Ketchum
LOVING YOU MAKES ME A BETTER MAN
You honestly felt that was true.

The Mamas & the Papas
DEDICATED TO THE ONE I LOVE
The ring I still wear.

Richard Hawley
BABY YOU'RE MY LIGHT
The first single you gave me.

The Doors
LIGHT MY FIRE
We came down the aisle to it – played on the organ!

Cyndi Lauper
TIME AFTER TIME
Played by Terry Wogan for you, from me,
when you were diagnosed with cancer.

Simon & Garfunkel
BRIDGE OVER TROUBLED WATER
You played this when you announced your cancer;
I cannot hear it without thinking of that moment.

Bruce Springsteen
IF I SHOULD FALL BEHIND
Encapsulates our caring for each other.

Judy Collins
AMAZING GRACE
Your final song on-air and at your funeral.

Joni Mitchell
BOTH SIDES NOW
Though you didn't know it when you were 'down here',
your coffin would come in to this.

NOW

GOODBYE, WOGAN HOUSE

I know I like everything neat, but it really is something to fall terribly ill on New Year's Day. It's made measuring time so easy.

Christmas 2023 is such a quiet one for us. We just have to make sure you don't catch anything. We avoid parties, and go out just one night to the Grosvenor Arms in Hindon. We sit at your favourite corner table, where you can hide your portable oxygen machine and wear your nose cannula without being too visible. We order pizzas, salad, red wine. We know how to date well together. Isn't it a great evening, just you and me bantering and quaffing away? 'You should live in Hindon when I'm gone, Duch. It would really suit you,' you say, glowing from the wine and the ambient warmth of the pub. Thank goodness it is such a gorgeous evening, for neither of us know it will be our last night out together.

On New Year's Eve you are doing your first live show at Radio 2 since the end of September. We both know you have declined since then, announcing as you did in early December that this would be your last Christmas on earth.

For six weeks you were muttering your concern about doing the show live. It will be your seventh live one of the year. Pre-records at home in your den have become a necessity due to your health. But New Year's Eve is an important day and all the shows are live that day – unusual for a Sunday. I keep saying that if you aren't up for it then Bob Harris would happily cover for you. Of course, you won't hear of that. It's one thing to have cover when you're away on holiday, but when you're in the country, no! Good old DJ paranoia. Seeing how worked up you are getting about it, I realise it will definitely be the very last live one, so it is laden with significance.

It doesn't help that we couldn't go to our flat in London the night before. You've long ceased to be able to get up the stairs, even though it's only on the first floor. That part of our lives has already been taken from you. From us. It means that we drive up from Shaftesbury in the morning. You drive. You love driving. You're the best driver I know. Fast, confident, yet safe. You love your Lexus. Such a workhorse of a car that has done you proud for fourteen years, taking you up and down to London. We arrive so early that we have time to drive up to Primrose Hill so I can go into the flat to collect the post and check it. You stay in the car. You want to follow your usual routine of driving past Pret a Manger on Great Portland Street and getting lunch. It's closed. I feel your heart sink. Although it is unspoken between us, we both know this will be your last live show. It's sad that your normal pattern is curtailed. No matter – a new Gail's has opened right opposite and in there I blow an eyewatering £28 on a couple of loaves, a sandwich for you and two small salads. It's our opening conversation in the studio with Paul Thomas, your executive producer – the expensiveness of Gail's. We sound like two country yokels experiencing the high costs of the big city for the first time. In fact, Paul and Jamie, the studio manager (SM), whole-heartedly agree.

You are on fire as you broadcast. The text machine goes nuts. Hundreds of messages pour in for two hours. Johnnie is live! Let's get him. I sit opposite you, sorting requests into piles – Bruce, Eagles, Bowie, Rod, Elton, Steely Dan, Stevie Wonder … All through the show the music choices are free-forming according to requests. You get your jingle and sound-effects package going. Car horns abound. You may be wearing a nose cannula so you can get enough oxygen, but who would know? Your adrenalin is pumping.

Tony Blackburn comes in for an impromptu on-air chat. The two of you are hilarious together. You give him such a hard time, basically telling him he's obsessed with himself and his own fame. Tony wittily responds, saying he signs autographs to himself. It's bloody funny. I know there's a one-off show between the two of you in the can to be broadcast in March, but honestly everyone missed a trick not putting you two together more often. Off-air, he asks why you're on oxygen. You lie, saying that you have a bit of a cold. I am quite certain that Tony is not fooled by that lame excuse.

As the two hours draw to a close you start making mistakes. I know you aren't getting enough oxygen to your brain. When I tell you that my dearest friend Jacquie is listening in the Seychelles with Gail, you give a name-check to Jacquie and Claire. 'Awks,' texts Jacquie on hearing it. 'Who is Claire?' Gail asks.

It's emotional for me, saying goodbye to Wogan House. For almost eighteen years you've been broadcasting from here. I take photos of everything – the studio, the mic, the control room, Elton's piano, the coffee machine. You are too far gone to be emotional. Being the gentleman you are, you spend some moments with Clement the doorman, who himself is a gentleman. It's all very poignant, walking away from a building that has been your longest-lasting broadcast home. All that history in there. The memories of so many guests and presenters soaked into the walls. The end of a big era.

We both know I will drive us home. I take us up Marylebone High Street with its Christmas lights. We pass Nottingham Street, which is where we lived for the first few years of our marriage, in the spacious, wonderful flat that I wish we'd never sold. As we go down the Marylebone Road towards the Westway to leave London the tears fall quietly down my face. I instinctively know that you will never come to London again and that over twenty-two years of fantastic fun that we have had here together has ended.

It's New Year's Eve. Across the country people are preparing parties and getting changed. We are tonking down the

M3 and A303. We are rewarded with the occasional burst of fireworks. You tell me I drive well – a compliment I always love because of your own skill. Your Lexus is the largest horse in our stable of three. It's like taking out a thoroughbred that's just a little too big and strong for me – but fun to ride.

As we approach home we weigh up our options. We can't drop in at a pub or restaurant because a) they will be fully booked and b) I think you will fall asleep. So we head home. I light candles, put out a cheese board and one of the Gail's loaves and open a bottle of very expensive red Burgundy, which must have been a gift from our close friend Charles. I do not realise the heavy symbolism of my choice. Bread and wine. The Last Supper.

We watch a few minutes of the New Year's Eve concert on the BBC. Slightly blurred from the wine, I go to my bath-room. I turn on the radio as I always do when I enter any room alone. Sat on the loo, I hear the midnight bells from Big Ben chime. I roar with laughter. This strikes me as the funniest way to see in the New Year. Loo flushed, I go to find you to share the hilarity. I find you in your bathroom, also on the loo. We both see in 2024 on the John …

New Year's Day, 1 January 2024 – the day our lives turn upside down. If it wasn't for the fact that we are due to spend it with Jane and Charles, you would have stayed in bed. They, d'Arcy, Gary and us – the gang of six – have so often spent NYE together. Once till 4.30 a.m. as you once bragged about on air. But because of your show yesterday, it has to be a New Year's Day lunch this time. You do look a little grey as we get in the car. I can see your energy is low. Once again I drive, neither of us realising that you have driven your last. Such a loss for you – you, who might have been a racing driver if not a DJ. You were training at Jim Russell's racing school in 1966 when you got a job on the pirate station Swinging Radio England, later jumping ship to Radio Caroline. DJing has certainly provided greater longevity than racing would have. Your destiny was to play tracks, not drive on them.

At Jane and Charles's, in front of their roaring log fire, you sit with your coat on, shivering. You look white. You cannot drink. You don't eat. You just shake. Getting covered in more and more rugs. When you go to the loo you make such a noise that Charles stands like a sentry waiting for you to come out in one piece. When you do, all you can do is cry on my shoulder and ask, 'Duch, what's happening to me?'

I left the key in the car. Somehow it runs down the battery. The Lexus won't start. What a day. Now dark. Jane drives us all home. Happily, she has drunk very little of Charles's fine wines. Sadly, so have I. You go straight to bed. I stay up and feel annoyed with myself that I agreed to a lunch today. I should have known that you'd need a complete day of rest after a show. What a start to 2024.

THEN

FALL AND I'LL CATCH YOU

You were standing in for Terry Wogan on the *Radio 2 Breakfast Show* for the two weeks after the wedding. We were high on love. In bed at every possible moment. It meant that our actual honeymoon had to be delayed until Terry returned. We chose Kerala in India, and I can only say it was the worst holiday of my life. I already had 'honeymoon cystitis', and somehow we just didn't take to India the way so many do. While the food was sensational, and the Ayurvedic treatments fabulous, there were many negatives. The mosquitoes were appalling – I was covered in bites even before we did the dreaded backwater cruise. In a small boat with a small crew, where it got dark at 6 p.m. because the sun sets so early and there was just one fading battery-run lamp, where we had no wine and had to huddle under mosquito nets, we endured what you always referred to as the worst night of your life. You wanted to jump off the boat and swim to shore, you were getting bitten so badly. While we had booked two nights on the boat, we begged to be taken back to shore in the morning. The dear crew couldn't understand why we weren't loving it. I almost had blood poisoning from the bites. Meanwhile you were going into yourself. You became more and more distant, telling me you weren't joining me for supper. You claimed to be feeling ill. I thought you were being tricky. I felt certain that you were regretting getting married. My abiding memory is sitting alone at dinner with my half-bottle of white wine. (There were only two wines in India in 2003 – one white; one red; both awful. The same brand wherever you went.) The entertainment provided was a young Indian man with a guitar singing 'Tequila Sunrise' by Eagles. The whole trip was so ghastly that I cannot abide that song, and I have never returned to India. I doubt I ever will.

The Delhi Belly you returned with continued for months. You finally agreed that you should see a doctor. However, you did not have a tropical disease as I thought. In fact, you had a growing obstruction in your bowel. While you said nothing to me, this had been your fear. It was with such guilt that you held my hands outside the private clinic only metres from our Marylebone flat and said, 'Tigs, I'm so sorry. I have cancer.' This was even worse to take on board than the cancelled wedding. *Oh my God*, I thought, *he's going to die.* Nothing had or has shocked me as much in my life. It was a Friday and so we were going down to my cottage in Ashmore for the weekend. Even though it was you who had been given the diagnosis, I was the one who fell apart. We had gone through so much turmoil to marry, just for you to then die? I couldn't fathom it at all. You drove the whole journey while I wept. It took all weekend for my shock to pass. On this occasion you were the strong one, calling your children, Sam and Beth, to let them know the terrible news.

You were a public figure on a massive weekday radio show – this was not something you could hide. Having told Radio 2 management the news, you made the announcement on air, playing Simon & Garfunkel's 'Bridge Over Troubled Water' for all those suffering with cancer. You stepped away from your show, and we spent the first year of our marriage together fighting the non-Hodgkin lymphoma in your bowel. It was such a rapid gear change to everything in our lives. If there had been any semblance of a honeymoon period lingering after India, it ended sharpish.

We hadn't lived together before we married, so this was a baptism of fire. We had recently done up and moved into a fabulous mansion-block flat in Marylebone. While I thought the flat would be a wonderful, positive fresh start to married life, it became a place of fear, stress and illness. You were so sick. Chemo knocked you about in a way I've never seen since. You were hospitalised between each cycle of the poisonous drug combination known as CHOP. I stopped doing any commercials. I existed for one thing only – to help you survive. I became cut off from family, friends and work. Later I would learn through our work with Carers UK that this is the norm. Carers become isolated. It's partly because you are caring, and partly because you just don't want to share your story. It's too hard for people to hear. Too hard to share. And feels almost disloyal if you do. You became my work: taking you to Barts Hospital at all times of the day and night; answering to your every need. I was slowly going inward, getting lost, getting nothing in return. If I thought I knew you when we married, I soon realised I didn't at all. You were so consumed with a fear of death that you became difficult and closed. On occasion, cruel. Indeed, more than once I thought I'd made a terrible mistake and married a total bastard. The more needy I became for reassurance, affection or gratitude, the more insular you became. It was hell.

During a few days at my Dorset cottage seven months into your treatment, you were rushed to Salisbury District Hospital. 'Call a fucking ambulance!' you shrieked in excruciating pain. After an afternoon on a ward when your life was slipping from you, you were diagnosed as having peritonitis. Your bowel had been perforated by the chemo. You were given lifesaving surgery in the middle of the night. You were on life support for the next few days. Visiting you when you were conscious again was the greatest relief of my life; you asked me to get on the bed with you, and your dedicated nurse left the room so we could hold each other in complete privacy. You always say that was the most overwhelming moment of love in your life. I wasn't as relaxed. I was terrified of pulling out one of the many tubes coming out of your body that were keeping you alive. It would have been ironic if I'd accidentally undone all the doctor's good work.

The surgeon, Nick Carty, said to me as you started to pull through that you were far from safe. He also added that you should never, ever smoke again. It was the worst thing you could do to your body. I took this message very much to heart.

After a month of recovery in hospital, when your huge, fourteen-inch-long, extremely deep stomach incision had to heal up, you had to learn to walk again. When you were released you returned to a new cottage in Farnham, Dorset, as I had moved home in your absence. You wanted a cottage with a garage for your motorbikes. I sold my beloved Clock House for you – one of several property moves I would later regret.

You named the thatched house 'Marky's Cottage' after a man in the village who had been born there and lived in the village all his life. His only absence had been during the First World War, which he'd fought in under-age. This was a promise you made to him in the pub one night – where you were instructed to have a Guinness a day to build you up. You'd had a few red wines too. So while you were a tad inebriated when you made your grand declaration, it was a lovely gesture and immortalised a true Dorset character and a part of the village's history.

You credit that cottage, its woodburning stove (which you sat next to daily), our new working cocker spaniel Fergus and the Museum Inn as your route to healing. Ultimately, all the chemo, surgery and care had worked. The following spring you returned to your *Drivetime* show, much to the delight of all. You had been off-air for just under a year. Meanwhile, in a parallel of our life, in the script I was writing, *ANTONIA*, I had the groom fall ill on honeymoon. I've never explained that to anyone, it's just my nod to the shocking start to our marriage that we endured.

You went on to have many more operations and illnesses. It's as if the cancer took your health and immune system down a big notch, because other problems crept in. I must confess that having given my all to you during your cancer year, my heart would sink when something else went wrong. *Oh, not again*, I would think, and sometimes say. I remember one stint in Salisbury District Hospital when I told the registrar that you had to be released because you were on-air at the weekend. He looked at me askance. 'But he has pneumonia. He's very sick.' Again, when you had been taken to hospital in an ambulance, I was beyond shocked to hear from the cardiac nurse who called the next morning that not only had you just had a heart attack, but that you needed a triple heart bypass. 'Can he do his show this Sunday?' I asked (I was by this point your agent and manager). Again, I was told, 'Your husband is very ill. He'll be off work for six weeks at the very least.' Over the years I visited you so often in hospital, taking you your specific requests from home: sweeties, food, tissues, clothing, batteries, radios, magazines, toiletries, DVD players … You saved your mischievous requests for others. As you waited for a date for your heart bypass, you persuaded a friend to bring you in a bottle of red wine. Goodness knows what others brought you. Fags? Jack Daniel's? Oh, how you enjoyed being a monkey.

The result of so much medical intervention is that you ended up with scars going all the way up your body, from your ankle to the top of your chest, as if you could be entirely unzipped. I've always joked that very little remains of the man I married, as it's all been removed, replaced or enhanced.

The one illness that did not leave an outward physical scar was the one that finally got you. Months after your triple heart bypass, which entailed them opening up your sternum and wiring you back together again, you kept complaining that they had retied you too tightly. You felt a heaviness across your chest and still found breathing diffi-cult. You wanted to be opened up again for them to redo it. Instead, the heart team referred you to the respiratory team. You were made to do breath tests on and off treadmills, you had scans, and then, in August 2019, we went to meet Dr Rohan Mehta from the respiratory department. He told us that you had idiopathic pulmonary fibrosis (IPF). In layman's terms, this meant that your lungs were inflaming, scarring and then being rendered useless. Idiopathic means that the cause of this was unknown. We learned that it was incurable and that while steroids and certain extremely expensive drugs could slow the progress, nothing could reverse it. You were given a prognosis of two to five years. I asked about a lung transplant but was told that would be plan D. Reading between the lines, you were probably already too old and too ill to receive such an enormously invasive operation. We sat in Dr Mehta's room, trying to quantify this amount of time. You were seventy-four. I was calculating how many more holidays we had left; you were wondering if you'd make it to eighty. Happily, you did qualify for the extremely expensive drugs that could stem the progression, but sadly you were one of the 50 per cent of patients who reacted extremely badly. Dr Mehta agreed that £10,000 a year of NHS money was not well spent if it gave you constant diarrhoea.

You bought a portable oxygen concentrator. A box the size of a cereal packet would hang over your shoulder on a strap, and a plastic cannula would provide good-quality oxygen through your nose. You could turn it up or down as needed, and you went everywhere with it, including Radio 2. You wore it during shows, and you soon wore it all night, which led to us parting to separate bedrooms. Later it would be replaced by a far larger and noisier machine that became your lifeline in the final year of your life. Life was about oxygen levels and heart rate. Steadily, you could do less and less, and I had to do more and more.

It wasn't just you who suffered sickness in our marriage. Ten years after your cancer interlude and five years before your heart attack and IPF diagnosis, it was my turn to call in the caring favour …

Of all the rollercoaster moments of our life, the one I will always consider the hardest is the one that I believe caused my breast cancer. I always bragged to you that I would never get the disease because I let everything out, but when something occurred that I could not discuss with a soul, I felt the tumour in me starting to grow. I will never forget the morning. It was a Saturday, and I had just returned from an early-morning walk up to Shaftesbury with our latest working cocker spaniel, Darcey. You were still in bed in our room at the Old Fox and Hounds. You said, as you did whenever some shit had hit the fan, 'Tiggy, I need to discuss something with you.' The tone of your voice and your use of my name gave away that there was menace behind the discussion. It normally took you days to summon up your courage to broach difficult subjects, but a gun was pointing at your head. The Jimmy Savile saga has put a slur on all DJs of your generation, but it also opened the floodgates for women to make accusations, and you were an obvious target. An anonymous woman in Manchester went to the police saying that you had sexually abused her in the 1970s backstage at a gig. She alleged that you had ripped her tights and groped her breasts. Somehow, the head of HR at the BBC and the latest controller of Radio 2, then Bob Shennan, had been informed, presumably by the police. By 11 a.m. that Saturday we were on a call with Bob, who said he needed to take you off-air. All I could see was your well-earned, incredible reputation – plus our life – falling from beneath us. Everything. Our entire identity. Destroyed. In one fell swoop. You didn't deserve such injustice. And despite that occasional little dark streak of yours, I know that fundamentally you always have been a very good, decent man – with a few character flaws. We discussed with Bob that if he took you off-air, it pretty much sent out a signal that you were guilty. The anonymous woman would have won before any evidence had even been heard. Bob, in his fairness, finally agreed. You could stay on-air, and the whole issue went to the Crown Prosecution Service (CPS).

You were interviewed within weeks, but when you heard the evidence you immediately smelled a rat. You were described as having buck teeth and curly hair, and reeking of whisky. Since you'd never had buck teeth, and curly hair was a brief post-chemo phenomenon much later in your fifties, and it was a well-documented fact that you detested Scottish whisky, the evidence was utterly flawed. What was correct was that you were at the said club the night she claimed, as you were the compere, but so, too, was a band, which included one member with buck teeth, curly hair and a taste for whisky, who has since been done for abuse against women. That didn't stop you being under investigation for months by the CPS. There was no case, the police who interviewed you immediately realised that, and the wait was intolerable. It was unfair, unnecessary, unjust. I felt the stress of this situation every second of my waking life. I held it, this ghastly threat. I believed completely in your innocence, but was utterly powerless. I felt my life force diminish. I discovered the lump two months into the waiting game.

My main memory of chemo, which I hated with such a force that I ended up needing talking therapy to get me through it, was me lying in the guest bedroom feeling utterly sick, my head pounding, with me crying my heart out, yelling, 'That fucking woman!' and you crying that you were so sorry that you had caused this. Fame – why do people want it? I felt so sorry for you. You always had an over-developed sense of guilt, and here I was, suffering deeply because of something you were falsely accused of. It really upset you.

I believe right down to the depths of my soul that the mistaken allegation of that woman caused my cancer and thus also destroyed my future health, for you never completely get over the threat of cancer returning. That fear is always lurking at the back of your mind. I was so angry with her that I fantasised – a lot at the time – about going to find her and confronting her. She hadn't hurt you; she had hurt another woman, an innocent sister. You were strong. You knew you were innocent and all would ulti-mately be fine. But I was not used to the machinations of being in the public eye. Never before had I felt the down-side of fame with such overwhelming force, and never before or since have I had to keep such an awful event in our marriage a secret. You've always had a favoured expres-sion: 'No amount of worrying ever changed tomorrow.' It's been a guiding light for you, that saying, and it has kept you grounded in your life of fame. I wish I had embraced that belief myself back in 2013. I have since reflected on the anonymous woman. I'm truly sorry she suffered sexual abuse. I too suffered from some in my youth, so I know the effects. I always chose to do nothing about it – it's all so long ago and would achieve little but pain for the remaining family of the man. But I do know this – time plays havoc with our memories and it is a deep sadness for me that she remembers the incident but not the perpetrator. I hope she has found some peace.

For the record, while you felt enormous guilt about my sickness, you really should not. The system failed us. The CPS was cruel and slow. You, my darling, were a steadfast and devoted carer. You took me to over seventy appointments, you waited, and you discussed at length all my fears. You held me as I sobbed with chemo sickness. You shaved my head when my hair started falling out. And for the only time in our marriage you put me before radio. Friends of yours could see your abject fear of losing me, but you never did open up to anyone. You just absorbed it, occasionally crying with me. Throughout that horrible eighteen months of operations, chemo, radiotherapy and Herceptin, you were my rock. I couldn't have got through that time without you. And should it ever reappear I don't think I could face it without you.

It was during this period that we became the co-patrons for Carers UK, a charity supporting unpaid carers. If only I'd known about them when I was caring for you; I would have coped so much better. Being a part of the charity gave meaning and purpose to our illnesses. Together we would go to events up and down the country, raising money and awareness of the need for support for the charity. We even took a group of friends to walk a section of the Great Wall of China – the wild section with uneven rubble, and no steps or barriers to stop you falling off. You struggled to get up there and I discovered I had vertigo, but an unforgettable week with the best views I've ever seen led to some deeply forged friendships and our group raising over £65,000 (a lot of which came from your friend, the comedian Peter Kay, who is a very generous man). I will always be proud of how devoted you became to the charity and all the good you did for them. Not just the Great Wall of China fundraising trip, but your willingness to attend all the events they held, being the star turn, giving talks, encouraging donations, meeting other carers, supporting the poetry events, talking about the charity on-air and being the catalyst to Radio 2 getting behind Carers Week. OK, I was the person motivating you and coordinating all these things, but you always said yes to everything the charity and I asked of you, and you really deserve recognition for that.

Everything really does happen for a reason and our health issues have meant that we gained such an understanding of what so many others also go through. You said to me from the start that you believe we are spirits on a human journey. The tougher it is, the more our spirits learn. Sickness and caring are two of the fastest ways to do that. So I guess it was worth it for our spiritual growth, as well as helping Carers UK.

MY TOP TEN
SONGS YOU SHARED WITH ME

Ryan Adams
LA CIENEGA JUST SMILED

Jackson Browne
FOR A DANCER

Avett Brothers
I AND LOVE AND YOU

Buffalo Springfield
FOR WHAT IT'S WORTH

Johnny Cash
HURT

Robert Plant & Alison Krauss
PLEASE READ THE LETTER

Lucinda Williams
RIGHTEOUSLY

Sixto Rodriguez
I WONDER

Josh Ritter
HOMECOMING

Nathaniel Rateliff & the Night Sweats
S.O.B.

FOR BETTER, FOR WORSE

We meet the palliative care nurse for North Dorset in November 2023, after a Zoom consultation with a doctor who said that it was time to get the ball rolling on end-of-life care. It was one of those throw-away comments that doctors can make without realising they've just blindsided you. End-of-life care … It's a medical catchphrase. You're asked, 'Is your husband receiving end-of-life care?' I don't know. Is he? Talk about a label.

Caroline Gullis is an angel in a smart grey suit and sensible flats. She has authority, wisdom, strength and empathy. I call her on 2 January 2024 and ask if I should be worried. And as it happens, she says that I should be. The days that follow are a blur of activity and change. She comes. She arranges others to come – district nurses, occupational therapist nurses, respiratory nurses, nurses I've never heard of, the GP. Your health has collapsed. Your lungs haven't collapsed but have taken a huge walloping. We are told that doing that live show was too much stress for your already very sick body, that you have no resilience and now can never come up to the level that you were on a few days ago. Your instincts had been right. You weren't strong enough for a live show. You now need huge levels of support and have been labelled a Gold Star patient. While it sounds like you've been promised a life of club-class flights, it means that because you are so vulnerable you now go to the top of the queue – for appointments, ambulances and any medical needs. These are your perks. Your priority status. Not that you wanted them.

A lot happens in six weeks. A lot. The fabulous local NHS set you up for your new disabled and nearing-end-of-life status. An occupational nurse comes to see what equipment you need. Grab rails? NO! Reclining seat? NO! Commode? NO! Stool for the shower? Well, OK. As it turns out, that seat is little used. Showering has suddenly become a hugely stressful event for you. Even though I'm there with you, holding the shower hose while you sit on your NHS white stool, with your nose cannula in, the steam makes you panic. You can't breathe. You take some of the many drugs you have been given to manage stress, but these don't touch the sides when it comes to the shower. It becomes an issue we choose to ignore: the fact that you are living life unwashed. It strikes me as letting go. A giving-up of the human spirit. We try you kneeling beside the bath while I wash your hair, but we end up at the kitchen sink.

The district nurses come in thick and fast – what a resource they are. When you are concerned about a new development I call them and they come round. Emma is your favourite. She has a wonderful manner with you. She plonks herself down on your bedroom floor and chats. She is calm, reassuring; she doesn't wind you up. It helps a lot that she used to be on a respiratory ward. Your greatest fear is that you are going to 'drown' from lack of oxygen and your lungs seizing up. She assures you that your body will just get more and more tired, that you will end up spending more time in bed, you will sleep more, and one day you just won't wake up because your organs are not getting enough oxygen. You take that. We both do. A gentle exit while you're in the land of nod is what we both hope for. Doesn't everyone? When, where, how? The moment of our death is surely the mystery event that we all think about, and in our sleep is definitely the favoured route.

The biggest issues are your oxygen and controlling the balance of your drugs. You've been given Oramorph – a liquid morphine – which helps calm you and so you breathe more easily. At first, I am terrified of you getting addicted to it, and I have grounds for my fears. I realise that every evening at around 6 p.m., instead of asking for a G&T, you are taking a slug of the new drug. The Oramorph Cocktail Hour. I suggest that it isn't recreational. You are defensive. Actually, you are rude. When I hide the bottle so you don't abuse it, saying I will give it to you when you need it, you go ballistic. We have a terrible scene. One evening when I'm already in bed you stagger into my room. 'Give me my bloody Oramorph.' Your desperation for it is deep. Your verbal abuse shocks me. I give you the bottle. Indeed, I throw it forcefully at the sofa next to where you're standing. I shout at you that my bedroom is my safe space, my alone space, that you must never come in there again. The huge sadness is that you almost never enter my room again. That was our last row. After that you are in charge of your Oramorph. I have to recalibrate. Stop being so worried. Your body, your stress, your survival method. We both have to get used to our new norm.

A week later the respiratory nurses arrive and assess your failing lungs. At this point you are still able to walk – not far, not fast – but their tests reveal the rapid rate of your decline. I am so alarmed by this that I say to them privately, 'He doesn't have long, does he?' They say, as does everyone whom we quiz on the length of time left, 'We cannot say. You just never know.' And they don't.

Two new large, loud oxygen concentrator machines arrive, with huge four-metre-long clear plastic tubes attached to them so you can move around relatively freely; long white tanks of oxygen that we rename the milk bottles; masks; cannulas … truly you are spoilt. Almost immediately you are on oxygen 24/7. The tubes become something I trip over – a health-and-safety hazard if ever there was one. One Sunday lunch in the future a tube will cause me to trip and drop a roast chicken on the floor as I bring it to the table. We still eat it – though the plate doesn't survive.

Despite your depleted state, you continue to make your radio shows. I let your executive producer Paul Thomas know what has happened. He is deeply sensitive, telling me

I must keep him in the picture because no one wants to push you too hard. They are remote, so they cannot judge when you should stop. That is being left to me. Liz Barnes, your incredibly patient producer, becomes even more patient. Of course, you want to go on broadcasting, but the shows start taking a lot longer to record. You get yourself to your den, I bring coffee and a Berocca, you print out all your notes, Liz appears on FaceTime and slowly you record the links. You lift your voice, digging deep. The links cannot be too long as you get breathless. 'Take your time, Johnnie,' Liz will say over and again. Some days the time you need to take is two days. You will do hour one on the first day, hour two on the next. It wipes you out, but you know that you have to keep going because if you stop, it's like saying you've given up, that the game of both broadcasting and life is over. This is one of those times when you reveal to me your inordinate strength of character.

Your voice is your livelihood. You know how you should sound, and you know that you don't sound like a robust Johnnie Walker anymore. The breathlessness cannot be completely hidden. That said, Paul gives your voice recordings a huge level of treatment before they are broadcast. These include a de-reverb plug to remove the room reflections from your den, a very heavy dose of AI noise reduction to reduce the wind sound from the oxygen concentrator, a 'soothe' plug to reduce any whistle from your teeth, some standard compression and 'limiting' to make sure your voice has broadcast energy, and finally a good bit of equalisation (EQ) to remove some of the 'mud' and put some air into the top end. You are now processed. Ultra-processed Walker. You are incredibly impressed by and grateful for Paul's extraordinary 'geekery'.

Radio 2 want to do a special retrospective show about you. Paul was going to come in December. If only he had; it would have been so much easier for you both. He and I get a date in the diary for as soon as we can in January. There is a sense of urgency between him and me to get it done as soon as possible. Just in case … I collect him from Gillingham train station. He is with us for the whole day, interviewing you in chunks so that you can have a breather in between. He is moved by seeing you in such a state. He last saw you in the studio on NYE when you were still able to strut – almost. You must seem so declined to him, and in just a few weeks. Paul has thought deeply about the songs you might choose. He almost nails it. He's done his research thoroughly and I can see he truly cares about you and the programme he's making. He's clearly very good at inter-viewing you, as he goes on to make a great tribute show. The end of that show makes me cry when I hear the final edit before transmission. While the three of us have lunch together you ask bluntly, 'Is this for when I'm dead or before?' The answer is 'both'. As it happens the reaction when it does play out at Easter is huge – and probably will be again when you're *brown bread*.

Paul is the first of many guests that start arriving. I find myself doing a lot of catering, worrying about what people will eat, trying to find time to get out and shop. I am suddenly time poor. You have gone from helping out here and there with the dishwasher and running the cars to being rendered totally useless domestically. What is more, I'm suddenly doing so much extra for you – early-morning tea and oatcake, two stages of breakfast, dressing you, emptying the pee bottle, making your bed, running around turning oxygen machines on and off as you move around, a lot more laundry as the new drugs affect your insides, juggling medical appointments and equipment arriving, washing your feet and your hair, organising and administering your pills, undressing you before bed, tucking you in, wishing you goodnight while wondering if it is the final time I'm wishing you goodnight.

The change to both our lives is dramatic, sudden and all encompassing. In the first six weeks of our new regime, I think you are going to die very soon. I certainly do not think you will make your birthday at the end of March. I cry every day. I am overwhelmed. I am struggling to cope. Fortunately, at this point very few people know you are unwell so contact from the outside world is as yet containable.

The thing I realise after some weeks is that part of my emotional breakdown is that I am grieving for our life together. It's anticipatory grief. We are never, ever going to go out anywhere ever again. I live for holidays, films and theatre, and going to restaurants – it's all I want to do. To go and do these things with you. And while, yes, you are still here with me at home, we won't ever do any of those fun things together. Ever again. It's unimaginable to think that our pizza together at the Grosvenor Arms in Hindon was our last date.

Jane, of the gang of six and my closest girlfriend in Dorset, is full of concern and wants me to go to the doctor to get an antidepressant. I think that would make me a failure. I am not depressed, I'm just not coping because I am overwhelmed. I resist for weeks. As it happens it is the greatest gift she has ever given me. I start them on 1 March and while the first four days are grim, by week two they start to make a difference. I am myself again. The Tiggy I used to be before I even met you. I feel like a survivor, not a victim. It's a huge step forward. I may never stop taking them! I am also offered counselling. I'm touched that there is such a level of care for the carer now. It wasn't like that twenty-one years ago when you had cancer. Nonetheless, I respond that I am fine. 'I am not depressed,' I stress, hoping that will be written in my notes. 'I am simply exhausted and overwhelmed.' I really couldn't pile having to talk about myself for an hour a week on top of everything else I have to do. Besides, I really don't want to leave you alone any more than I have to.

To get up and down the corridor from your room to the sitting room is getting so hard for you. You have to sit down after ten feet to regain your breath. It's painful to watch. You have been assessed and told you can have a wheelchair, but there's a wait. We have a mobility shop nearby in

Ludwell – Freedom Mobility. I go in there and find a treasure trove of items for the elderly and infirm, from wide slippers with Velcro fastenings to mobility vehicles. They have a wheelchair they rent out for £5 a day. A new form of car hire for us. I take a photo and share it with you. You agree it's a good idea, though I can see there's resistance in you. It's a step, isn't it? A step towards being less able, less of the virile man you have always been. It would just be there for back-up, I suggest.

I pick it up just after I collect your Australian grandson James (son of Sam) and his girlfriend, Holly, from the train station on 7 February. They have come to London for two weeks to stay in our Primrose Hill flat while we still have it. James was a teenager when we last saw him five years ago; now he's a young handsome hunk of a man. He brings in glamorous Holly and the black wheelchair as he arrives. You greet James warmly and within seconds jump into your new chariot – and that's it. Never again will you walk anywhere. The difference it makes to your life is massive. And how different our home looks as I roll up all the rugs decorating our wooden floors.

Something wonderful happens with James's visit. Your daughter Beth, James's aunt, wants to see him too. Because we can only cope with James and Holly staying one night as you're feeling so bad, Beth and her partner, Rachael, come to supper at ours that night. I do a traditional roast chicken and all the trimmings. We have a great dinner. You, unbelievably, pull yourself up the way you do for a show, regaling everyone with great showbiz stories, delighting James and Holly, and amusing us all. There is laughter, joy and love. Oh, the power of good food and wine! It is a night many of us will remember. The final time your family break bread together around our table, and probably the final time you will hold court with such aplomb. I'm so happy you gave James that memory of you.

The wheelchair is a blessing for you, a curse for me. You need to be pushed everywhere. I am well and truly house-bound with you in case you need an urgent trip to the loo. I feel the tension rising in me. I am dressing you, nursing you, pushing you. I feel stress quite keenly. I am on edge most of the time. One afternoon I need to pop to Boots for a prescription – thirty minutes, tops. I return to a sitting room in chaos. 'What's happened?' I ask, bemused. You needed to pee. You tried unsuccessfully to move yourself in the wheelchair. The result was a car crash, an accidental repositioning of furniture and you having to use your water bottle as a receptacle. After that we order a new pee bottle and I try to get the ball rolling on an electric wheelchair.

What a difference the electric wheelchair, 'Quickie', makes – to both of us. Because you love driving, you turn circles and go up and down the corridor. We both feel a sense of freedom. How you love to nip down to your den to do prep on your radio shows, or nip over to your table to get a box of tissues. You nip a lot. I just have to swap over your oxygen machines if you go from one end of our long house to the other. Each time I get the full blast of the piercing, hateful *BEEEEEP* as the new oxygen machine offensively and loudly switches on. And then the constant drone of the motor. Conversely, when I switch the machine off it shudders and comes to a blissful, silent halt.

Your boss Helen Thomas wants to visit. You are the reason she's at Radio 2 as you brought her in from Radio 4 to be your *Drivetime* producer. Your connection goes deep, especially for her. She loves all her presenters, but without doubt she has a soft spot for you as you were her first at Radio 2. She's always credited you with increasing her music knowledge. I have a new routine of collecting visitors from Gillingham station, bringing them back and making lunch while they chat with you. The car is a great place for Helen and me to have an honest conversation. We like and respect each other a lot, but we don't always agree. I say to her that you don't really have an ego. She snorts with laughter, saying you so do – that all her presenters do. They wouldn't be presenters without it. Well, maybe that's true, but I do think yours is under control and is one of the reasons you are so loved. I reflect on a recent conversation with Bob Harris, who called to see how I'm doing. He's been put on standby in case you stop broadcasting. 'When Johnnie stops are you getting the gig, Bob?' I ask, being nosey and territorial.

'Oh, I think so, don't you?' Now that, to me, is a healthy presenter's ego. You wouldn't say that. You wouldn't even think it. You have humility running through your veins.

Helen's visit is lovely. From the moment she comes through the door she brings in her fantastic energy and I see you respond. I realise that what you love to do now is reminisce, and you two have so many stories and laughs to share.

Before she leaves I ask if she wants a photo of the two of you together. She is thrilled. She's also incredibly photogenic. Of the many visitors we are to receive over the coming months, Helen's visit stays with me as one of the most special because, after me, she probably knows the real you as well as anyone else, and has been so instrumental and supportive in our lives. In the car going back to the station I touch her arm. 'Are you OK?' I ask, concerned. I'm glad I took that photo. It's hard for people saying goodbye to you. You've been a truly significant person in her life. I know that when I return home you will be exhausted, but relieved and happy to have seen her. I am right.

A commode. Your mother died on one, and recently your sister fell off hers and subsequently died. There's no two ways about it, you are damned resistant to having one in your room at night, but after an accident, as you can no longer rush to the loo, I suggest the time is right. You are deaf to my suggestion. Then one day, when a district nurse is visiting, I come into your room to find her sitting on your bed talking very sensitively to you. She looks up at me and smiles, telling me you have agreed to one.

I feel a sense of embarrassment when it's delivered. To the man dropping it off it's all part of the norm. For me, it is a sign of further decline. A nudge closer to the end. He shows me the locks on the wheels. The bucket underneath the plastic removable seat I discover for myself, which – I will later learn to my cost – needs to be pushed very firmly all the way in to protect the carpet beneath. You deny its existence and will not let it in your room. For some reason I park it in the guest bedroom, which also acts as my study. I have to avoid Zoom calls in there.

Its arrival is shortly before I go away on a recce to Sardinia for my film. I have to go and see the Mamuthones festival, as I've written it into my script without having experienced it. I have no choice but to go now.

Have I ever cried as much as when I leave you? I cannot speak the word 'goodbye' as I am sobbing too much. I am convinced I will never see you again. The pain is so great, the fear so deep, that I cry for over an hour in the taxi. The poor driver.

I have created a full schedule of the people who will care for you while I am gone. Our friend Claire, former godmother of Darcey Dog, has offered to do the overnights. She arrives each evening to find that a different set of friends has been round to bring you dinner and get you pissed. It's party time every night I'm gone, and Claire picks up the pieces. But she also does something else rather magical: she brings the commode into your room at night. She takes the fear and shame away. Together, you rename it 'the Alien'.

Reading the papers every day on your iPad as you do, you furnish me with all sorts of news that I don't get time to discover while I'm away. There is one piece of news that delights you. There's almost a sense of pride behind it. 'Do you know what you have done?' you ask me. 'You have put Vinted into profit for the first time.' This is a fact you share gleefully with every guest who comes round over the next few weeks.

It's true. Since you only wear jogging pants and incredibly casual wear these days, it struck me that some of your formal clothes clogging up both your and my wardrobes were surplus to requirement. You said you'd never wear them again, so they should go. And thus, my market stall began. It started with your dressing-up gear – the ghastly Seventies-style shirt and waistcoat that you wore at the Goodwood Revival festival when they recreated a radio studio in which you DJed. They go quickly. I move on to any lace-up trainers, since you can't do laces any more. Many of these are unworn and lucky men around the country are suddenly wearing almost-new HOFF trainers for a fraction of their original cost.

As you lie in bed I stand by your wardrobe pulling out individual items. 'Keep!' or 'Go!' are your commands. You are very certain in your choices. The goers are removed to my study and hung up on my stall. I photograph them, upload them to the app, put in the relevant info and off they go.

Offers come in. 'Duke, someone wants to offer £20 on the cowboy boots.' You are part of the process. You give a yay or nay to offers, and we find this hilarious. When we get to the really flash items you get more interested: the tailor-made three-piece country suit; the Barbour jackets; the Paul

Smith linen suit. Some I find hard to part with as I wrap them in tissue. None more so than your Richard James teal corduroy velvet suit. I think it is the best item you have ever bought. Richard James himself sold it to you in his Savile Row shop. My description reads: 'OK, peacocks – this is the best suit I've ever seen my husband in. Just style and gorgeousness in abundance.' I put it on for £140 – a big price on Vinted. Several men are in touch for exact measurements, sad that they are just too big, short or fat for it. It finally sells for the asking price to a man who sadly gives no feedback. Maybe he's a dealer and sold it on to someone else for considerably more. I hope wherever that beautiful bit of schmutter ended up, it is loved. I still miss it.

When my stall is empty I return to your wardrobe. 'You'll never wear this again,' I say, holding up a brown Gant cord jacket. You agree and make other suggestions. You suggest things that I'd have given to the charity shop, like a Stone Roses T-shirt – and you are right. You have a great sense of what has value.

Part of this is amusement, part of it is lightening our load so we feel less encumbered with 'stuff', but for me it is getting things done and sorted before I am grieving, when I won't see any joy in Vinted. In a way it's me preparing my path forward. If I sort this stuff now, I will have more time to grieve. When you become an experienced market trader on Vinted you quickly learn several things: get the price right; photography is key; women don't buy, they just like. Men are fantastic decisive buyers; sell to them at weekends

– they're bored. Package nicely. Despatch immediately. Putting in a note always goes down well. Labels sell. Non-labels are much harder to shift.

One weekend I make over £500. It brings us enormous amusement. In a pretty small life where you cannot leave your own four walls, this connection with the outside world seems fun. I keep telling you that we're sharing the love of all the beautiful, stylish clothes you have bought over the years. For, yes, my Duke, you have always been considered by my friends a snappy dresser and a darned good clothes horse.

In two months I take £1,327 – 90 per cent of which comes from your clothes. It's the start of the booze fund at your wake – a fund you consider very important, as you really want our friends and family to enjoy your send-off.

I've earned a night out. It's mid-April and I'm starting to suffer from cabin fever. The perfect excuse is needing to write a column for *Dorset Magazine*, and for that I simply HAVE to attend a talk by food writer Angela Clutton at nearby café Sorelle. I invite my friend Annabel to come with me. 'Stay out as long as you want,' you assure me. I prepare your supper and leave it out for you. I am possibly the most excited person at the event – I am OUT! – but the talk is over by 8 p.m. I'm crestfallen, so I suggest to Annabel a drink at the Grosvenor Arms. I let you know, and not only are you delighted that I want to stay out, but you ask if I can bring you back a margarita. This is the oddest request, but I'm used to odd requests from you. The bar girl, wanting to make you happy, asks her manager, but sadly they are not allowed to sell take-away alcohol. You look at me appalled when I return home empty-handed. I notice your untouched supper. 'Where's my pizza?' you ask, disconsolate. Never before have I twigged that a margarita/ margherita can be both drunk and eaten. It wasn't such an odd request after all, but you are disappointed, which I make worse by finding the misunderstanding incredibly funny. You do not at all. I make a note that you need a take-away pizza – soon.

THEN

HERE COMES
THE WEEKEND

I feel I met you too late. Of course, I met you when I should, but it came right at the end of your radio peak. I knew you for just your final couple of years on *Drivetime* (and you were off for almost a year of that). It was an incredible show, exactly what the BBC should broadcast. It had intelligence, warmth, entertainment, good music and a fabulous magazine approach with business news, sports, traffic and a daily guest. People would say how they would sit in their car in their driveway to hear the end of your interviews because they were so good. If an author came on, by the end of the evening their book was number one on Amazon. The influence and effect you had on your 7 million listeners was amazing. I loved watching you at work. You were a master in the studio, in total control, fully understanding what the listener wanted, what questions you should ask, what to play next, and of course all the knobs and faders. Masterful.

While I know it was hard on your energy after the cancer, with you staying in bed until the afternoon before going into the studio, you were still doing great shows on what had been your slot for seven years. When you drove down to our Dorset cottage one Friday evening in 2005 to tell me you were being taken off *Drivetime* you were devastated. Completely and utterly. It was just about the worst bit of news you received in our time together, second only to the cancer diagnosis. Not only did you love that show and your connection with the listeners, but you knew your peak was over. The controller, Lesley Douglas, needed you to make way for Chris Evans. Chris is a very clever, creative, energetic broadcaster. But he wasn't you. And ironically, you told me it was the second time in your career you were being fired to make way for him. It felt like Chris was your nemesis, and you found it hard to feel anything but blatant annoyance towards him. (No wonder I was uncharacteristically icy with him when we met a year after he had taken over *Drivetime*. I was actually told by Bob Shennan, the new controller, to go easy on Chris, that it wasn't his fault. I was quite amused at the thought of such a huge presenter being affected by me, the loyal wife!) Your dream, if you don't mind me sharing, was that you would get the *Breakfast Show* when Terry Wogan stopped. You did three months a year as cover, and you LOVED it. How you enjoyed giving people a positive start to their day. You would get all the team to stand at the window just before 7 a.m., open your arms and make a daily affirmation: 'We open our arms to all the abundances the universe has to offer …' and off you would go with a brilliant show. What we didn't know was that Chris had been brought in to Radio 2 specifically to take over that show when Terry stopped. A double whammy. You were collateral damage of management decisions.

Without a doubt, for you, me and millions of listeners, it was the first of many decisions Radio 2 took that upset its traditional, and extremely loyal, older audience. You always said, the glory days of the network were when Terry got people to work, you got them home, and in between Ken Bruce, Jeremy Vine and Steve Wright did fabulous shows. But times move on, and the management direction has been to attract younger listeners and be inclusive of female presenters.

It took you at least five years to get over the upset of losing your beloved show. You were moved to Sundays – the worst day of the week as you can't enjoy Saturday evenings, and so the concept of the weekend is pretty much taken from you. And business still takes place Monday to Friday – pluggers, requests for appearances and dedications, plus interviews for the show – so it feels like there's never a break or a down day. When at the start of 2019 you were given the *Rock Show* on Saturday nights it really was curtains for any sort of normal social life.

I would come up to the London flat with you to keep you company (having shifted our life to Dorset after you came off *Drivetime*). I remember the evening you struggled into the flat after 10 p.m., leaning on the big retro radiator as if you couldn't manage any more steps into the flat, saying this was no way for a man in his seventies to live. You were exhausted.

While Sundays started with a lame attempt at a spiritual show, in 2006 it became *Sounds of the 70s*. It was sad that your old friend and Cockney Rebel frontman Steve Harley lost that gig to you, but as he was always indebted to you for launching his music career, he bore no ill will and your friendship continued until his untimely death. It was a great decade for you to do, even though you had always hankered after the Sixties show (Bob Shennan astutely asked me if it was the decade you wanted or the time slot – Saturday morning). It upset you that you weren't playing new music, but as one of your former producers, Paul Rodgers, said, it was new music to the younger generation. It played to your strengths and knowledge, but with it something died in you – that desire to find new music that you could share on-air. You'd always been so proud of that – and so respected and known for that.

It wasn't long after you lost *Drivetime* that an envelope arrived from Number 10. 'If it's an invitation from Tony Blair, we're not bloody going.' It was, in fact, an invitation to receive an MBE. You didn't have to think about it. You knew your parents would have been proud, and mine still could be. And they were. It's very special to go to Buckingham Palace to receive this honour. Sam, Beth and I all attended with you. The then Prince Charles shook your hand and said, 'I suppose you're all going out for a jolly good lunch?' And he was right – we had a great one at Elena's L'Etoile in Charlotte Street. To my recollection that's the only time the four of us had a 'family' event together, as not long afterwards Sam and his wife, Jules, moved to Singapore. This was such a sad loss for you. Not only were you losing your 'son and heir', as you liked to call him, but your grandson, sweet baby James, too.

We took a major decision about our lifestyle at this time. You were finding London too noisy and busy, and suggested we move to a big house in the country. 'Are you sure, Johnnie?' That question again. I said how we could never afford to return to such an amazing apartment in London again if we left. You were sure. Absolutely certain. Yet when we sold that beautiful flat in Marylebone and bought a much smaller pied-à-terre near the BBC, *and* a bloody great farmhouse in Dorset, you weren't sure. You spent as much time as you could at the new London flat, agreeing to interviews any day of the week to have an excuse to be up there. I, meanwhile, was floating around a large – and haunted – five-bedroom house, wondering what the hell I was doing there and feeling very at sea. Once, as you were about to drive back to London, I even ran down the drive and lay across it so you couldn't leave. What did you do? You stopped the car, laughed your head off and took a photo of me.

It was while I was at that house, alone, that your biography came out in 2007. It was possibly because I was unhappy or because the ghost, 'Old Sod' (a name we learned from the previous owners), was giving me a hard time, banging doors at night, that I fell ill. I got flu – real flu – and was bedridden for two weeks. When I felt strong enough I opened the copy you had dedicated to me and started reading. Oh my God, Johnnie, I was horrified. Your life consisted of one situation after another when you trashed it. That reel-to-reel recorder you spent months saving for when you were a teenager and then threw it out of the window. Your rebellious nature at work; walking out of amazing jobs because of the music policy; living in a car with Sam when he was a little boy because you had no money. By the time I got to the part when you met me, I just thought, *WHAT have I done?* If I'd read that book first, I would not have married you!

You were unable to come home and look after me while I had flu, as there were important people to interview, but you were concerned enough to arrange for your friend Angela Donovan to come down with her husband and another friend, supposedly to give me a healing. I couldn't understand why it would take three people to get rid of my flu, and when they arrived, Angela walked into the room with an extraordinary hunched gait, like the Hunchback of Notre-Dame. I couldn't think what was up with her, but it turned out she was channelling Old Sod, the ghost! Within minutes I found myself sitting with you and those three, taking part in an exorcism of our house! Really, as events go, this was up there with the most extraordinary. I was totally freaked out, and then you all said you had to go. 'Johnnie,' I begged, 'please don't leave me. PLEASE.' You said you had to, you had an important dinner in London, so you lit a fire in my snug, told me to wait in there and promised me you'd be home by 2 a.m. You all left and, disconsolate, I went into my snug. The window was shut, the fire was lit – and there on my desk was a huge black crow, crowing. I have never been so scared. There was no way on God's earth I was staying in that house – we sold it six months later.

Next, we moved to a beautiful converted granary surrounded by fields. However, it was east of Salisbury, far from our patch in Dorset where all our friends were. The big lesson we learned there was that friends (and good pubs) really do make a home. We were like fish out of water. There was one upside – apart from getting our puppy, Darcey, and meeting Sarah, who became our right-hand woman – we were much nearer to Radio Solent, the local BBC radio station for Hampshire, Dorset and the Isle of Wight.

You asked me to call the controller there to see if you could have a look around. Part of you hoped that you might be able to do some of your Sunday shows from there to save driving up to London so often. So I called the managing editor Mia Costello, who seemed only too delighted for you to visit. We had a great chat on the phone, and she asked if I would come too. We were duly shown around their studios, and given the full guest-of-honour treatment. Just as we were about to leave Mia leaned over to me and said, 'You have a great voice for radio. I knew it when we spoke on the phone. It's why I wanted you to come.' Instantly, she offered us a two-hander weekly show! You were delighted, and I was flattered. When I put this to the then controller of Radio 2, Lewis Carnie, his response was immediate:

'Johnnie is a radio legend. He is NOT doing local radio.' You were annoyed, of course, but Mia took the news on the chin, and instead offered to train me up.

The Radio Solent *Breakfast Show* presenter Julian Clegg was given the task of showing me how to run a desk and speak into the mic, and before long I was doing stand-in on the *Early Breakfast* shows. It was fabulous to have the opportunity, but oh, how AWFUL it was to get up at 3.30 a.m. to be ready to take the station on-air at 5 a.m. How do people do that every day? I would get many texts from you, of course, giving me your expert tips. 'Put your fader up! Speak louder! Come out of the song now!' It was such a rock to have you there. The other thing you taught me was 'doors to manual'. For you, there had to be a way to get out of the set programmed music and put on a CD of your own choosing. You made sure I knew how to do that. I learned then that you and I have one big similarity – we are both obstinate about our music choices. After all, why do it if it's not for sharing the music you love? In the end I did twenty-five shows, both in the week and on Saturdays, which were later and involved a newspaper review, which was much more fun. Honestly, we were always so grateful to Mia for giving me the opportunity, and very sad when she moved on some months later, as the new man in charge certainly did not want Johnnie Walker's 'missus' doing any shows on his watch.

Our next move in 2009 was to Shaftesbury, back in our beloved Dorset, back near our friends and favourite pubs.

And there we stayed, doing up one house after another. By this stage you were used to your weekend working. You had found your new rhythm and had finally got over the upset of coming off *Drivetime* and not getting *Breakfast*.

A number of years later, in 2018, I made another foray into radio, and when it came to my voice behind a mic you were nothing but complimentary. You loved it. So when I told you I'd got myself a weekly radio show at community radio station Abbey 104 in Sherborne, you were delighted, and when it went out you were actually impressed. I've always liked a magazine-style show, as you had on *Drivetime*. I played great music because I could play whatever I wanted. (Not being cocky, but you always loved my taste in music. It was slightly different to yours – a bit younger, certainly – but good enough for you to pick my brains each week for ideas for your own show.) My magazine features included a weekly arts round-up of TV and film, a guest interview – you and Leo Sayer being my top two bookings – and 'Tiggy's Kitchen'. I really believe in spreading the word about home-cooked, healthy food, so each week I would cook a dish at home and then get you to try it, recording as I went. While you weren't exactly Stanley Tucci in your praise, you did generally react well to my efforts, though a few months in, when I created an okra sensation, you just went 'Yuk!' on tasting it. How we laughed! It was great radio.

I loved doing that show. I had listeners around the world (thanks to being your wife), and the great thing is, they stayed with me for the entire year that I did it. The show was called *Afternoon Delight* and, yes, my opening jingle was the corny song of the same name.

A year later, in 2019, one thing that could happen because of your weekend shift was the *Sounds of the 70s Live* tour. This consisted of you talking about the decade, interspersed with live renditions of some of your favourite songs of the decade. Leo Green was the musical director, and Damien Edwards the lead singer. It was a great show, and the audience loved it, but your health was fading by then, having already been diagnosed with IPF. You had been on intravenous steroids for a week to give you strength, but all it had done was bloat you (and led to me cheekily re-naming you Bloaty McBoatface). The band also did Tony Blackburn's *Sounds of the 60s* tour. We would hear that Tony was dancing every night and doing combat rolls on stage. Really?! It was all you could do to sit on a stool and make it to the end of the evening. After the sixth show you lay on the sofa in your dressing room. 'Please tell me that was the last one.' I had to break the news that there were sixteen more. It was too much for you. Your sister Maureen came to that show, and in her firm, big-sisterly way she said to me, 'He's not well. He needs to take care and slow down, or else …'

In the background, fans from Scotland and the North were complaining that you had no dates up there. You felt bad about it, but you just weren't well enough to do such long journeys and return for your weekend shows. This was not something we could say publicly because everyone in showbiz has to keep up the impression that they are fit, well and ready to broadcast.

You had various well-respected agents during our time together, but none of them brought you any extra work. You were never comfortable with TV as you were afraid of the camera lens seeing into you, plus, by your own admission, you were bloody lazy. So they didn't have much to work with. The result was that, as my commercials producing career had ended, I could support you and became your agent and manager. I was free, and though I say so myself, I am an amazing scheduler and full of ideas. On the one hand this was a brilliant solution. On the other, it wasn't. My life became focused around you, your career and trying to keep you healthy. At meals we would talk shop. Our life became the business of you and your diary: you being on-air, you doing interviews, you doing talks on a Saga cruise, you attending this or that, you doing tours and shows.

Without any doubt, the successful career girl I once was had taken a step back. I was now the main support for the Johnnie Walker show. And while I enjoyed learning about the radio world (and doing some myself), my own creative and financial needs were not met. Where once I had earned more than you ever did, now I took a small stipend from the business. Of course, you always said, 'Pay yourself more, Duch,' but you never were great at financial realities. No longer did I buy designer clothes or go to fancy restaurants – but in all fairness, nor did I need to. What I missed was the excitement of a new creative project and working with my production team and crews, feeling I could make a real contribution in my own right, not just as the back-up crew to you.

My father would reassure me that I was doing the most important job that I could. 'Behind every great man stands an even greater woman' and similar platitudes would flow from him whenever I complained to him privately about my lack of fulfilment. To my father you had an enormously important role in society, making millions of people happy. As he saw it, it was a greater use of my time and skills to keep you going than making commercials to sell things people didn't want or need. He was a wise man who believed in duty. 'What can we do for others?' seemed to be our family motto.

My mother, too, was always concerned that I was looking after you. When once I said I was going to New York for the weekend she simply replied, 'But what about Johnnie? Who's going to look after him?' It was incomprehensible to her that you could survive alone for four days. Indeed, she herself took this responsibility to heart. Where once I had been the central character and driving force in my family, I was gradually pushed away. No longer did my mother want shopping days with me or a day out to an art gallery. She'd always say, 'But, darling – you're SO busy,' and without me even realising it, a huge separation was occurring. I was so conditioned to be a good wife, to put my needs last. Indeed – to have NO needs. I feel I was the last of a generation of women who did not demand their own rights to a career or freedom. I admire and almost envy the women of the generation after me. I mean, I didn't even have kids, I just had you! But somehow a life in the public ear and eye is demanding. And you had already been so ill. Alone, you weren't great at coping. We both knew that. Just think back to how you lived in that terrible flat when I met you. As I always say, you were my destiny, and I know I kept you broadcasting for many more years than you would have done without me. This gives me comfort and an understanding of my decisions. That said, I will never marry again. I'm just no good at it. I mean, I am good for the man. I'm brilliant! But I get lost at my own expense, and I never, ever want to do that again.

I ran every element of our lives, business and domestic. You just had to do the shows. (And even then, you'd ask me for song suggestions!) You were as happy as Larry. You didn't have any stress. I did. When we had an almighty six-year fight with HMRC about IR35 (the off-payroll working rules) I spent much of my nervous energy dealing with our accountants, lawyers and the BBC to get it resolved. It was only in 2023 when I sent my accountant a letter stating that you were now under palliative care, which he shared with HMRC, that they finally backed down. After many thousands of pounds of fees, and a lot of time and effort, that particular nightmare was over, but the fact is, I have done a lot of fighting for you. A lot.

So, for balance, let's remember something particularly wonderful about being involved with your career:

lockdown. The most magical few months of our marriage. Not only did it give me the perfect reason to cancel the remains of the *Sounds of the 70s Live* tour, but also this time most certainly extended your life, as you no longer had the exhaustion of schlepping up and down to London each week. Everyone over seventy was banished from BBC Studios as a safety measure, so you now had to do your show from the garden room of our beautiful Georgian farmhouse that we'd renovated in St James, Shaftesbury. You called your friend Rodney Wayman, who lives locally and had a business in recording equipment – Solid State Sound. He ran to your rescue, getting a RØDECaster mini production studio and mics set up.

Coincidentally, you also fell terribly ill at that time. You had already been diagnosed with IPF the previous summer of 2019, but you were so ill that, with the sense of medical panic across the country, it was assumed you had the dreaded Covid already – which in those first weeks was considered a death sentence. The GP told me to call your respiratory consultant, Rohan Mehta, and ask if you would be put on a ventilator if you went into Salisbury District Hospital. At that point a ventilator was considered the only hope for Covid survival. While he was hugely sympathetic about you being so ill, he was honest, which I will always be grateful for. He said you would not be put on a ventilator. My guess is that younger and healthier patients would be put on them long before someone in your already weak predicament. You would be put on a CPAP machine on a small ward, and I would almost certainly never see you again. I was gulping down uncontrollable tears.

I called the GP again. This time I spoke to Dr Perkins. 'Look, what if it's a chest infection?' I argued. 'Why don't we just stuff him with antibiotics just in case?' She agreed completely and within the hour a volunteer was at our front door with the drugs. When I took these to you I spoke in no uncertain terms: 'Johnnie, there's two lots of antibiotics here and you are going to take them all, no questions, because right now you are fighting for your life. Understood?' You nodded compliantly and opened your mouth. As it happens, Dr Perkins and I were right.

However, you were too knackered and ill to do your show alone. Knowing that you had successfully thrust me in front of a mic on the *Radio 2 Breakfast Show* a couple of times, and that I'd done my summer of *Early Breakfast* fill-ins on Radio Solent, as well as my own weekly afternoon radio show at Abbey 104 for the previous year, you felt safe with me sharing the airwaves with you. You asked Lee Thompson, your then producer, if it would be OK to use me on this one show. Lee said it would be fine. Good man! No one asked Helen Thomas, who was now the controller of Radio 2, because you knew she would say no, so you just did it – you and Lee, dicing with the management. After the show went out you called Lee to ask about the reaction. He was amazed. There were even more emails than usual – everyone had loved me being on with you! So we did it again, and again. You loved it. Lee loved it. The listeners loved it. And I loved it. But one person did not. Helen. We were given the impression that she hated it. You say it was because you never asked her; she says it was because the format of the *Sounds of …* shows is a single presenter. It was the one big stand-off you and she had, but it could not be argued; at this extraordinary time, we were replicating the locked-down lives of so many people around the country. You claim I made you speak in a different way – I was your bounce, as Sally Traffic had once been – and it is no exaggeration to say that you adored having me on the show. We recorded the links on a Tuesday, and I gave up each of those days, helping you select songs, requests and subject matters. I would prep the room with blankets and cushions to soak up the sound, which would later be treated by executive producer Paul Thomas with his computer 'add-ons' to improve the quality of your voice. Lee was brilliant with me; he gave me the reins but didn't let me slip up. And you, Johnnie – nothing was ever better than doing radio with you, the master. I was like Darcey Dog looking up to you with awe and respect. You were the top dog, and I was next to you, wagging my tail. Happy, happy days.

However, the fact that Helen wasn't happy meant that all was not well. A phone call with her had me in tears. 'I love you, Tigs, but this is *Sounds of the 70s* and you don't belong on this show …' she told me. So after five months, during which I had worked for absolutely nothing yet felt I had made a big contribution to lockdown, I stood down.

You were very upset that I stopped, feeling that the show lacked something without me, and you really disliked going back to pre-records alone. If it wasn't this show, you really wanted to do another one with me – as Mia Costello had suggested years before. 'They spend their lives trying to create on-air chemistry with presenters – and failing – yet we have it in spades,' you said. Oh, you were angry. We did a few specials together for Boom Radio, but the prize you were after was the BBC. We both knew it would never happen, so I say, let's be grateful for those five months. To this day I have people telling me how they loved it and how much it improved their lockdowns. And that, for me, is *almost* gratitude enough.

One great result of doing these shows was that I was contacted by Helen Stiles, the editor of *Dorset Magazine*. She said she liked my 'voice', by which she meant the things I said, not my diction, so this was when she asked if I'd be interested in writing a monthly column for her magazine – 'I can't pay much but I'm lovely to work with.' After the first column about us doing the show together, Helen gave me the lead columnist's position, just inside the back cover. She will never know what a boost that was for me – not only me finding my voice again, but just having something to focus on outside of you. Calling my column 'Life's for Living', I now had an excuse to experience all sorts of things in Dorset and write about them, but more than anything, my relationship with Helen became one of great importance to me. It was a lifeline outside of 'us', and she was absolutely right: she has always been lovely to work with.

Our radio stint also led to us doing a series of podcasts together. Northern Irish producer John Daly said he'd love to do something with the two of us. The best idea we could all come up with was that we as a couple should interview other couples, and as I have naturally developed quite an obsession with the person behind other thrones, I loved the idea. John came up with the fabulous title, *Consciously Coupling*, and Hotel Chocolat agreed to sponsor the show to promote their Velvetiser hot chocolate makers. Then we just had to find the right couples. These days everyone with a name is asked to be on every podcast, or so it seems. Usually there is no fee, but Hotel Chocolat, being the decent, ethical company that it is, sent every couple a Velvetiser and a selection of their hot chocolate sachets. Not a bad sweetener!

The interviews mainly happened during the second and third lockdowns, by which time we'd all accepted the quality of Zoom interviews. For us, it was fabulous just to commune with other couples, as we were all so starved of socialising. I was really pleased with the cross-section of guests we had – such a variety of relationships. Clare Balding and Alice Arnold were our first couple; they were delightful, warm, natural and so obviously meant to be together. Plus, Alice had been Clare's carer through cancer, so we had mutual empathy about that. Recording in the early evening, it felt as if we should all have a huge G&T in our hands. I really wanted to meet up with them afterwards and felt I could easily slump down on their sofa for an evening.

Hairy Biker Dave Myers and his wife Lili was a totally different story. She was strong, almost critical of him, while he simpered, amused by her power and soft insults. You asked if she had been afraid of the *Strictly* curse when he had such a memorable time with his dance partner, Karen. Lili looked at you askance: 'Have you seen him in Lycra?' Dave clearly adored her, but I would say she wore the biker trousers.

Damon and Georgie Hill were lovely together, so honest and warm, navigating a life where he was well past his Formula 1 driving years and now presenting. It felt they had come through a lot together – like Georgie's fear of him crashing – and got to a place of calm and deep support for each other. Anton Du Beke was as we expected: hilarious, an entertainer, scarred by his childhood but finding solace in showbiz. The story of him meeting gorgeous Hannah was hilarious, and she laughed delightfully and supportively most of the time. Fellow radio man Ken Bruce with his wife, Kerith, were emotionally the closest to us. I think only you radio men know what it's like to go in day after day and perform no matter your mood or circumstance. They talked openly about caring for their special-needs son, and their warmth and love for him and the family was wonderful. They were very natural, good, honest people, and I felt we got a rare glimpse into Ken's true self. We did twelve really different couples in total, and were often asked which was our favourite episode. It's fair to say we liked them all. Just like parents with their children.

These podcasts scratched your itch, but I would say without doubt that apart from not being asked to do *Desert Island Discs* on Radio 4 and not getting the *Radio 2 Breakfast Show*, your major radio disappointment was that we never had an official radio show together. You knew that we would be great. You knew that we both loved the banter and that we had great chemistry together on-air. It would have been fantastic, and I know we would have made people happy, as we did on the few Boom Radio shows we did together, but it wasn't to be.

After lockdown, when you were allowed access to BBC Studios again, you returned to Wogan House quite a few times. One notable stint was when Tony Blackburn was ill and you agreed to stand in for his *Sounds of the 60s* shows early on Saturday mornings. Very early. I came with you to each one to give my support and hated that alarm going off at 4 a.m., but you were a pro and just got on with it. You really enjoyed doing these shows. You love Sixties music, and the sense that your day was done by 8 a.m. was invigorating. You also appreciated the energy in Wogan House on a Saturday morning. You saw your old mucker Sally Traffic each week and Dermot O'Leary would pop in for a chinwag. So different to a Sunday afternoon, when often the shows either side of yours were pre-recorded so no one else would be in.

It was on one of these Saturdays that you inadvertently took a black sweet out of your mouth and left it on the side of the faders, as you suddenly had to speak. You were always fastidious about leaving a studio spick and span – all rubbish thrown away, cables neat, chair in place – no one more so at the station, I would imagine. So when I heard Michael Ball the next morning, shocked and appalled that someone – a presenter – had left a black Jakemans sweet on the fader, all hell broke loose. He was naming all the possible culprits – Zoe Ball, Rylan Clark, Liza Tarbuck. The one person he said it would not be was Johnnie Walker, because he was far too professional. Presenters called in to plead their innocence, and the mystery for Michael was intense. On hearing this, I went into you, still in bed. 'Duke, is there any chance that you left a Jakemans on the fader yesterday morning?' Your hand went straight to cover your mouth. Your eyes widened. Ashamed, you realised that yes you had. You immediately texted Michael, who received the message while still on-air. To his great shock, *you* – the only one he was sure was innocent – were the guilty party. 'Jakemansgate', which lasted almost an entire show, was solved. Later, when you went to the studio for your *Sounds of the 70s* show, you bumped into Michael holding a bag of Jakemans. His face in that photo was priceless. You just looked like a naughty boy, laughing. Walker, you were caught!

Once Tony was better, your executive producer Paul Thomas shared an idea: to record a show with both you and Tony. A musical face-off: the Sixties versus the Seventies. Everyone liked the idea, and later in 2023 it was recorded. You each took turns to drive the desk, and obviously whoever was driving had the power. I came in for the final half-hour of the recording; you were in the driving seat, and I couldn't believe the stick you were giving Tony, who in return was firing back reposts. 'Oh my God, he's being so rude,' I said to Johnny Kalifornia, who was producing.

'That's nothing. It's been fireworks for two hours,' replied Johnny. I was inwardly concerned that you had been too vicious, and I think you worried about the same, admitting that you gave Tony quite a hard time – I did not envy Johnny having to edit that one. The result was 'Clash of the Pirates', and it was without doubt the funniest radio show I have ever heard on Radio 2. I've no idea if it got any awards, but it truly deserved them – for you, Tony and poor Johnny K, who had to make it broadcastable.

It's a shame that you and Tony didn't do more shows together. Two true radio legends, two pirates – so different in style, but the affection, shared history and respect between you both has always been palpable.

GOING PUBLIC

You seem to have plateaued again. You go down a notch and you stay there until something pushes you down to the next level. During these plateaus we get accustomed to our new normal and adjust our actions and expectations accordingly. I feel safe enough to make a suggestion: I want to interview you. I want to capture this time while I can. You're a radio man, and your voice is your greatest form of communication. I feel deeply that you have things that need to be said, which cannot be said in a Seventies or rock show. That you have thoughts, wisdom, experiences, beliefs that should be shared. I think your listeners would be interested in knowing you better. You agree.

I have a first stab at interviewing you in your den, but you're a bit tetchy. You are an instinctive and brilliant interviewer, and because you find it so easy, you tend to be critical of my interviewing style. 'That is TWO questions. Why are you LOOKING at me like that? What are you trying to ask?' Crikey, you can be tough. On the second attempt I get better answers, but you do seem a tad breathless. I wonder if you are finding this stressful. It's only after twenty minutes that I realise I have failed to switch on your oxygen machine as we came down the corridor to your den. You contain your annoyance at my dreadful nursing, but it doesn't stop me feeling very bad about it.

I dwell on the recordings and realise it's going to be quite a tough edit, especially as the best bits are so breathless. Nevertheless, I am sure there is something usable and interesting there. I call John Daly from OJO Productions, who made our podcast series, and share my hunch that you should be recorded talking about this time. Something tells me it could be of interest, because you are now counting down your weeks and months. It's a profound time and, being the spiritual man that you are, it is surely a poignant and reflective time. I ask if my interview could go up on our podcast site and if it would cost anything. 'It would cost you nothing,' he says in his charming Northern Irish lilt. 'And what is more, if you'd like me to come over [from Belfast] and interview you both, I will. If it would be helpful.' It is such an instinctive, immediate, heartfelt offer. You agree with me that it's a lovely idea. We've only ever known John on Zoom, so just from a purely social aspect it would be great.

I collect John from Gillingham station on 11 April 2024. We chew the cud together first and then set up in your den around a small table. I've no idea what we will talk about, except that I know caring should be part of the discussion, though by no means exclusively. I am alarmed when you start proceedings with a question for me: 'Can I ask you something? … As soon as we returned from honeymoon in India I was diagnosed with cancer, so the vows of in sickness and in health were immediately tested. Now, here we are at the end of my life, when you're having to care for me all over again. You definitely saved my life when I went through cancer – I'm positive I couldn't have made it without you – your love was just so sustaining and gave me so much to look forward to, and your caring for me now makes my days so much better than they would be without you. Do you feel life's been a bit unfair to you, that you've been landed with this person who's required so much care?' My answer is immediate: 'It's been a long journey of caring. I think that's made me wiser, more compassionate, more patient. I think it's been one huge great learning curve.'

I've never been interviewed by you before, but I rather like it. You get straight in there, disarmingly so, demanding an honest response. John sits beside us, quietly listening. He interjects with small questions, gently guiding us down a path. He and I both make sure you don't talk too much, as you quickly run out of puff. He stays the night at a local B&B, not wanting to impose on us. He is a remarkably sensitive and kind man. The next day we record more, and you go off on quite an obscure spiritual angle. The difference between me and John is stark: I say, 'What the hell are you talking about that for?' while he says, 'That's great,

Johnnie. That's great,' knowing full well he won't cut it into the finished programme – he's keeping you positive and engaged. He knows how to handle talent.

We are exhausted after John goes but pleased we did it. He leaves with hours of material, and I feel very glad that he is editing it and not me. I wouldn't know where to start or end, as it was such a broad conversation. When he sends us his first cut a couple of weeks later we are amazed by what he has done. We only mention one thing we would take out. He then drops in music that Fergus Thirlwell composed for our podcast series. It sits in there so well, providing wonderful, delicate punctuation points.

Together we agree that the perfect time to put this on our podcast platform is at the start of Carers Week, on 10 June, but first I suggest that I send it to Helen Thomas at Radio 2, in case she'd like it for BBC Sounds. You say she'll never go for it, and I agree, but John and I both think there's no harm in asking. You are a much-loved member of the Radio 2 family, after all. Helen is a busy woman; the WeTransfer link runs out and I assume nothing will happen, but then, as she goes to a D-Day celebration on a train, she asks for a new link. She listens, and within twenty-four hours not only has she heard it, but so have all the management team at the network. They would love to mark Carers Week and put it on BBC Sounds, with Jeremy Vine topping and tailing it and three songs you spoke about dropped in. They don't want to change a word. They all think it's amazing. I get emails from all the station bigwigs saying how incredible it is. We are most of all thrilled for John and his OJO production company. He gave all his effort, time and travel for free. Now this was being rewarded by having a far larger exposure than our podcast platform would achieve. Over the ten podcasts, we had around 160,000 listens; the scope on BBC Sounds would be so much greater. On top of that, Radio 2 get behind Carers Week wholeheartedly. The entire thing seems to have been blessed with fairy dust, like nothing else I've touched before. A lot of people hear it (the BBC don't release podcast figures, but we are told it was 'a lot', and honestly, everyone we ever meet subsequently seems to have heard it). The social-media posts about it certainly get more likes than I knew possible. Even if we don't quite understand why, people have found it moving.

'HELLO?' I say unwelcomingly, even angrily, down the receiver of the house phone. It says *Anonymous* on the screen. I don't want to speak to them and it's a very bad moment to call, but I feel I have to answer.

It's a bad moment because a very old pirate radio friend of yours has been calling all week. Whenever I've picked up the phone to him he's announced himself with such self-congratulatory confidence that it sounds like he's going to tell me I've just won £5 million on the lottery. 'Hey, Tiggy! It's Keith …' I cannot handle him, not right now, which is why I've ignored the constantly ringing phone all day. Lisa, my hairdresser, has just arrived – she's doing you a favour, coming in after work to cut your locks. You're being slow and truculent in your room, struggling to put on a T-shirt. 'I will not be hurried!' you yell at me. We are both so frayed at the edges.

Yesterday I was on the Jeremy Vine show at Radio 2. Being the loyal co-patrons of Carers UK as we are, we both agreed that letting the world know about your IPF in Carers Week would help highlight the plight of other unpaid carers. While you've secretly had the disease for almost five years now, these past six months have been on a different level, and we feel that something needs to be said, to explain your ever-shortening links on a show if nothing else.

I was so calm when I walked into the new Radio 2 studio. I love a radio studio for its quiet, still, cut-off-from-the-world space. The way the heavy door closes with a gentle whoosh, shutting out any outside noise, sealing you in, safe. Jeremy was so warm, his hug full of love and concern. The headphones on, the microphone almost at my lips – I felt I could speak gently. I don't really know what I said to him. It just came out, from my heart. He got you on the line, and I pictured you in your wheelchair, your oxygen on Level 9 – it's highest. You sounded dreadful – panting, hoarse, struggling. I am so used to your voice, but hearing it coming down the line into the studio where I was and you should have been got to me, and I started to cry quietly. As Bruce Springsteen sang 'If I Should Fall Behind' (the live MTV Unplugged version) you cried too, as did many listeners. Jeremy came to sit next to me, and Ryan the producer brought in tissues. We continued the conversation, and you were completely on point regarding Carers Week. So very you – not wanting to be the focus, thinking of others, embracing the caring brief and ignoring Jeremy's more personal questions. Nonetheless, Jeremy had a moment of epiphany when he realised you will never come to the station again and that he will never see you again. I could see it hit him.

Messages started coming in immediately to my phone from friends who had no idea how ill you were. I answered them all the way home on the train and have been all day today as well. I balked when Radio 2 sent me the Instagram post they had done. I was filmed and had no idea. Thousands like it. I wish I'd worn more make-up, but I'm pleased I wore my blue linen jacket. The things we see that others don't.

When we sit and make these grand decisions to speak out we forget about the fallout, how overwhelmed by attention we will be. It's as if our energy is stolen from us. All I could do on my return was lie on the sofa. It was a Monday night, but we had red wine with some cheese for supper. I couldn't cook. Not last night. I was spent …

You are just coming into the kitchen, your T-shirt finally on, heading to the sink so I can wash your hair before Lisa starts cutting. My sleeves are rolled up, the big white jug full of warm water. I know it's difficult for you having a hair wash because you have to stand for over a minute – you have to work yourself up to it – but your hair is so filthy, and Lisa is still quietly waiting.

The phone rings at just the wrong time, but what if it's something important? I am always warm when I answer. Today I am not. I am stressed. I am exhausted.

'HELLO?' I say, my voice telling the caller to fuck off because they are a nuisance and have chosen the worse second of the day to call.

At the other end a calm, kind voice responds: 'Hi, Tiggy. It's *Elton* …'

I bluster. Try to apologise. Get my knickers in a twist and give up. I hand you the phone and you and Elton John chat away like the two friends of old that you are. Your lives have gone down very separate paths, but Elton wants to make sure he thanks you for all you did for him (like help get his first number one with Kiki Dee – 'Don't Go Breaking My Heart'). You in turn thank him for a truly beautiful deed he did for my brother Simon. Simon was one of the leading goldsmiths in the country, working for Theo Fennell. He made masses of jewellery for Elton, and when he was dying of cancer you asked if Elton would send him a message. You meant a short text. Instead, a video arrived of Elton telling Simon how talented he was and how grateful he was for all the treasured items he had made for him. In truth, Simon saw this on the last conscious day of his life. You upped the ante somewhat and told Elton he saw it in his last hours. Well, it was close enough. And for Simon it was one of the greatest accolades he could have received at the end of his extraordinary career. Elton is a good, kind man, and how typical that you felt you had to give him thanks rather than receiving it.

None of us is perfect, but I am a complete house snob – I don't mind admitting it. I grew up in a beautiful timber-framed farmhouse in Hampshire (which my parents bought for £15,000 in 1966). To me, it was the norm to live in houses with character and draughts. Throughout our marriage I've done up a number of places and I have loved doing it, every house demanding a different approach. Our previous house was a beautiful, small Georgian farmhouse on the edge of Shaftesbury. I remember the day I first drove down St James Street and noticed it. I nearly crashed it was so beautiful. Instantly I knew I wanted to live there, and about eight years later, after an enormous and expensive renovation, we did. I loved that house. I was proud of it. It was our forever home. With the help of my interior designer nephew Mark Lewis, we did a great job – it was even featured in two house magazines. It's also where we did our five months of *Sounds of the 70s* together. Fond memories …

However, it is also the house where you first fell ill with your lungs. Was it the house? The damp patch that appeared above your bed? The porous nature of stone? Or just bad timing? Whatever it was, it became increasingly difficult for you to walk upstairs. You had to sit in our bedroom chair to recover each time. Your den was on the top floor of the house, and you never went there as it was such an effort.

I realised with a sinking heart in the summer of 2020 that we were going to have to move again – just five years after moving into our 'forever' home – this time to a house with a downstairs bedroom and bathroom. I scoured Rightmove and noticed a development of three one-storey houses being built down the road in Hartgrove. At our first viewing it had a roof and breeze-block walls, but that was all. Taking a huge plunge, we put in an offer and put our house on the market. In December, we swapped Georgian character over three floors for characterless modernity over one floor. It is the greatest gesture of love I have ever shown you. And for you it was the perfect house to move into. Warm, well insulated, and not one step to be found. I would joke with you that if you ever needed a wheelchair, you'd be fine. Your health instantly improved, much to the amazement of your respiratory consultant.

While the house has an impressively huge open-plan main room with vaulted ceilings and incredible views across the rolling Dorset hills up to Shaftesbury, it just is not a pretty house. If I drove past it – which I wouldn't, as it is so tucked away and private – I would almost certainly say I never want to live there. But you love it. You've never been happier in any of our homes. While I have always felt that the house I live in is a reflection of me and part of the definition of who I am, for you it is more functional. In fact, I will go as far as to say I felt ashamed of it when inviting people round. Yes, I AM a house snob. Hands up. Guilty.

So it is the greatest irony of my life that we have never

had more visitors to any house than we have had to this one. And I have never felt as ashamed as the day our friends John and Steph Illsley came over. Their house on the Solent is one of the most amazing homes I have ever been in. It epitomises everything I might once have hoped for: large, relaxed, full of art, homely yet stylish, amazing jaw-dropping views over the water. You can feel the years of family living that have happened there; happiness and contentment drip off the walls. But then John is the bass player of one of the most successful bands ever – Dire Straits – and not a BBC DJ.

As they arrive one Friday afternoon in April, I hear myself apologising for our gaff. I want to hide I feel so ashamed of our modern rabbit hutch. I wish they were visiting our stunning Georgian farmhouse, but that reveals such an insecurity in me. They agree it is the perfect house for you, and they are fabulous guests. Steph arrives with such beautiful goodies: flowers from her garden, a yellow glass vase, sensational homemade cheese biscuits from her mother, Daylesford biscuits … All such thoughtful and perfectly selected offerings. What I love about their visit is that John sits close to you and gets right in there, asking how you are. He is so caring. Why shouldn't a rock star be like that? I am just very touched by how gentle and kind he is with you. And Steph is so warm with me. This visit goes deep into my heart. Steph later writes that they loved their visit and would love to pop over again. It's a lesson for me. Maybe I am not defined by the house I live in.

I have had a policy for the past couple of months that if you want to come and see us for supper, you bring it. Jane and Charles, our besties, came last night, but she too is caring for her ninety-six-year-old mother and just didn't have the time or the culinary joy to make supper, so I suggested fish and chips, which I know they enjoy. We had never had fish and chips at home. You thought it was a great solution, and I was ecstatic when I collected them – £46 to feed four of us, and all I had to do was drive into Shaftesbury. It was an adventure. Despite our limitations, there are still new experiences to be had. Charles brought two bottles of Chablis Premier Cru because he knows it's my favourite white, and because he is a very generous man. Always.

This takeaway experience will not be repeated – our delicate stomachs cannot take it. How glad I am that I persuaded you that 'the Alien' (your commode) should be parked next to your bed last night, stomach-churning though it is for me to deal with this morning. But sadly, it's part of the caring story. Your pee bottle is easy to handle; the commode bucket less so. It makes me retch. But I love you. And I know you feel embarrassed. Possibly ashamed. You mustn't.

Shall we talk about sleep? The fact that as you get more, I get less. You're on about fifteen hours a day to my five. Bedtime is two hours earlier than it used to be, but the summer sun rises early. It's not just the light that wakes me; it's also the wildlife from living in such a rural setting – magpies, a distant cow that wants milking, a cockerel. To add to nature's disturbance, you seem to need more early-morning visits to the loo. You have a thing about the Alien – your mother dying on hers goes deep – so you'd rather climb into your wheelchair and go to the bathroom. You yourself are quiet, but the *beep-beep* and *whir* of your vehicle drives me to distraction. And because you enjoy a bit of precision driving, you go backwards and forwards, backwards and forwards, often getting tied up with your oxygen tube. Tomorrow I will tell you that you HAVE to sleep with the Alien in your room again. *Every night*. We have slipped back from Claire's great triumph in February. You love to get your way, and not sleeping next to it is your only request each bedtime. Now it's no longer negotiable. I'd rather deal with cleaning it than be woken by the noise of you in the corridor. While I respect your neurosis about commodes, I'm afraid I'm playing hardball on this one.

There's something about sleep deprivation: it turns you into a grumpy, self-pitying victim. Oh, you're dying, are you? Well, what about the fact that I've not slept for days? What about me? I'm not a jealous person, but your ability to sleep is beyond enviable.

In my desperation for a proper kip I take a sleeping pill, temazepam, illegally given to me by a friend. I wake eleven and a half hours later. I don't know when I last felt such bliss. I could have slept even longer, but it's a big day. I've actually slept past the call telling me that your hospital bed will arrive in an hour. I have to get you up. I tear the bedding off your small double bed. As I manhandle the mattress and divan into the corridor, a sadness hits me that you will never sleep in a normal bed again. *Another last*, I think. I replace this sadness with a self-congratulatory pride that I managed such a physical job alone and even have time to hoover.

It has been quite a campaign from the nurses for you to get this bed. They think you will find it easier. It has a wonderful selection of controls: you can raise the whole thing up and down, tilt up your back, raise your legs or do both of those at the same time and turn yourself into a sandwich. The mattress is plastic, but I put a padded cover over it so you don't even realise when you get in it. I fear a reaction from you, but you seem pleased. Indeed, you go back to bed as soon as you've recorded your *Rock Show*. It's a licence to rest all day, and you can, you know. Tilt up, tilt down, sleep – eat your heart out. I've ordered a table so you can eat in bed with greater comfort, and so the hospitalisation of our home continues.

I've followed many a diet during our marriage. My propensity is to curve; I'm a juicy pit pony of a girl and have had very few moments in my life where my body was looking good, despite exercising and always eating healthily. One of the things I love about this period is that we are on the 'Keep Johnnie Happy Diet'. I'm pathologically unable to cook unhealthy food, but I have been allowing carbs and I'm trying to cook foods you actually enjoy rather than feel you should eat. I mean, when I went Paleo I did feel for you. The most exciting life ever got was a sweet potato wedge with your white fish and greens.

I am loving this freedom, and the strange thing is that I have lost some weight – but that is probably because I am running around more, or because of the sertraline antidepressant I'm taking. Or perhaps it's the new breakfast regime. You are eating so much less, but I seem incapable of serving you tiny portions. I know that eating and breathing together is hard, but let's be honest, your appetite has shrunk. You eat so slowly, and you look at most dishes I serve you for about thirty seconds before starting, as if you're thinking, *How the hell am I going to attack this?* I sit opposite you feeling guilty for asking you to eat something when it's so hard, even though I have cooked from scratch and with love. Food can heal, but not in your case. You leave a good portion of your plate, and because I grew up in a family of eight where nothing was ever left, I save all your leftovers for my breakfast. Today I am having one spinach falafel, with tahini and crudités (from yesterday's lunch), plus a helping of a courgette and butter bean dish that was last night's supper. An odd combination to kickstart the day.

Today is Wednesday. A great day in my week as Mariana, our cleaner, now comes for an extra couple of hours so I can have a guilt-free morning off. Today, tennis, and meeting a friend called Jan who lost her husband to motor neurone disease last November. She cries every day still. I cannot imagine how awful that must be. I absorb this with dread. As you note over lunch, 'Well, you won't cry every day.'

'You're right,' I agree, 'I won't,' and we both laugh. The truth is, I've no idea how many tears lie within me, or for how long they will flow, but I really couldn't keep it up for that long. Poor Jan. I'm glad she has her sons to comfort her. I wish I had some children who would comfort me when the time comes.

When Claire Allfree from *The Telegraph* interviewed us last week for Saturday's paper I joked with her about post arriving addressed to Johnnie Walker DJ Extraordinaire, Dorset. 'Please don't write that,' I asked. 'We'll be inundated.' She did write it, and now we are being inundated. The pile builds up for you to open. Credit HAS to be given to the wonderful postal service of Dorset – they never make a fuss about it, they just deliver. They read the messages such as, 'Please, please, lovely post people, deliver this to our National Treasure. Thank you.' The British are so polite. And they send such beautiful wishes. You mean SO much to your listeners.

Another thing Claire wrote is still smarting with me: that we sleep in separate rooms. Yes, we do, but I read it as if we are romantically separated, when in fact it's because you sleep with an oxygen machine that is so sodding noisy that no one knows how you sleep next to it – but then you are partially deaf. I sometimes try to cajole you into my bed for the night just so we can hug, but you like your room, and close proximity to your machine. I miss the skin-on-skin touch. The closest I get is when I bathe you, gently letting you down into the water on your bath lift, but only my hands touch you, lathering you up and rinsing you down.

The fallout from an intense week of publicity is with us. Whether you have been exhausted by it or just feel relieved that your truth is out there, you have gone off into one of your distant, dark places. You are and always have been 90 per cent light, but your 10 per cent of dark will sometimes rear its head, as it has this week. You close yourself off, go into your computer world, shopping for things you don't need, going down rat runs of conspiracy theories and goodness knows what. You shut me out. Your hearing is getting worse – that doesn't help. This week we've been two ships on different routes. We've not even passed in the night. The culmination of you being lost is always that you smoke. You struggle not to, because I am so against it for your health. Unfortunately for you I can always smell it when I come back home. You feel guilty, I get upset, you become defensive. We both know it's indicative of how down you are. It's your smoke signal that you're unhappy.

Smoking has been the reason why I have thrown my wedding ring at you more than once. I've even gone away for days. I just cannot understand why you would do that to your body when so many people have fought to help you live – not least me. You know it punishes me, and maybe that's why you do it, but more than that, I know it's your 'fuck it' action. You just don't care. You want to be drawn to the dark and not the light.

It was only Angel Caroline, your palliative nurse, who made me truly understand that you are an addict, and I can never change you. I now accept that I cannot. It doesn't, however, mean I accept that smoking is a good idea, given the state of your lungs.

As I've been lost, exhausted and angry this week, I have withheld my full-on caring powers. I've only done the perfunctory jobs for you, like meals. For two days your pee bottle has not been emptied, your bed has not been made, or breakfast delivered to your bed. I have not spoken to you except when necessary. You know you've hurt me, and because I am tired of caring, tired of being tied to these four walls, tired of putting you before my career, tired of carrying the whole damn show all the time and never having any fun, I feel used. This is my protest. While I do it to show I'm hurt, I wonder if it's also an oblique form of punishment.

I remember a medium called Jean who I spoke to last year. When I ask for another reading, the first words she says are 'housebound' and 'France'. My father appears. He is adamant that I need a break, that I am being taken for granted and not being given anything in return (he's changed his tune in heaven!). Jean says I *must* take a holiday at the end of July, that you should go into a home and I must not feel guilty. I believe Jean is right. It has given me the freedom and permission to think for myself for once. I mean, I had thought that you would be long gone by now, and yet you keep going. Jean says your body is weak, but your soul is strong. She's not kidding. She says your soul is stronger than mine – yup – but she cannot tell me when you will go, even though I ask. She would have to talk to your soul, and she is not allowed to do that. All she will say is that they're preparing a lovely garden for you up there. Keep up the digging, I say. I share with her my fear that you will outlive me, that I will keel over from exhaustion or get cancer again. She says that I must tell my soul that cannot happen. It's a warning that I take seriously.

Afterwards, I listen to a message from my friend Camilla. Would I like to join her and her mother at a house she's been lent in Saint-Hippolyte-du-Fort in the South of France at the end of July? It's uncanny. My flight is booked within hours and now we just have to work out what to do with you.

When I tell Angel Caroline she agrees it is a very good thing for me to do. Respite: I need it – her words, not mine. We discuss what to do with you. I mention that you've been smoking, and it is the first time I hear this calm, controlled woman sound horrified. 'Not in the house?' she asks, alarmed. I don't know because you do it when I'm not here. 'He mustn't. There is so much oxygen in your house he would explode. He must be off his oxygen for at least forty minutes and he must be outside.' She really is afraid of you self-combusting. I mean, there is a funny side to this. A cartoonish end. A headline if ever there was one: 'Johnnie Walker DJ Explodes!' Departing as a human firework – you never do things by halves. Just try not to take the house out with you.

I hope that the thought of a break from you will give me the strength to get through the next five weeks before my trip. I'm starting to pack my washbag already I'm so excited. Freedom, travel, planes, stimulation, friendship, laughter, baguettes, local wines. No caring duties at all. Never has the word 'respite' sounded so sweet.

We need to really make sure that whatever time we have left together is loving. I think a break from you will help that from my side, and I hope from your side too. I mean, it probably isn't normal or right for a wife to ask her husband if he is ever actually going to die, as I did this week. It was cruel of me, but it comes from you being cold and me being terrified that you will outlive me because I am so exhausted. I get paranoid about chest pains. I feel trapped. I can't go on like this forever; I do need my own chapter to start. I cannot stress enough: I was certain you'd be gone by now, but like the Duracell Bunny, you just don't stop. I ask myself – I ask you – 'What are you holding on for?' You seem to be indestructible. Great for your listeners, not great for me. Do I strike you as unloving? Or just very angry that you now take so much and give so little? You have an excuse now, but it's always been a bit like that. Unconsciously, I signed up for that when I met you, but right now, the balance has tipped even further, and we're in a place that is hard for me to stomach. I think and hope that this is because I am just overtired. The break cannot come soon enough.

You lie on the sofa and ask me to sit by you. You take my hand and tell me it's getting harder. You suggest that the game may soon be up. I am wary. I tell you that you have told me that before and then pulled back up. It leaves me on an emotional roller-coaster, and I ask that you bear that in mind, but maybe you are sharing your fear. I do understand that. Without doubt we are grappling with not knowing the when or how. The mystery of death is hard to contend with – in my case because I cannot plan; in your case because you must be wondering just what the hell is going to happen. My fear is that I am being too practical. I do the Waitrose online order and wonder if I should get you more digestive biscuits and cornflakes knowing I don't touch them, and if you should suddenly go, they'll go to waste.

Every single morning I go into your room and check to see if you're breathing. I often delay going in, in case you are not. What will I do? Who will I call? Will I just want you to myself for a final few hours first, before all the drama and bollocks start? The next chapter in our show. Will I regret the final words I say to you? Or will I need to tell you then, too late, how you have been the biggest, most extraordinary thing to have happened in my life? Too often I tell you how many sacrifices I have made to keep you on the road. Have I told you enough what you have brought to my life? The excitement, the fun, the amazing companionship, the love, the incredible lessons you have taught me about strength, chutzpah and belief. Have I told myself that? Or will I only realise when it's too late?

MARTHA AND THE VAN DWELLERS

I know that if anyone asked you what you loved best about being married to me, it wouldn't be sex, drugs and rock 'n' roll. It might be our homes, the stability and the laughter, but I suggest it would be that I got you travelling in a way that you had not before. Yes, you'd had plenty of motorbike trips in France and America with your mates, which fed your wanderlust, but for you it was the journey, not the destination. I flipped that around, broadening your horizons, getting you to enjoy the places we stayed in. And you loved it.

Honestly, for someone in showbiz you really had not tasted much of the good life. Wild, yes, but not what I considered good. Radio, I soon learned, is the poor relation of the media.

After you were so ill with your cancer, I booked us three weeks in a friend's hotel in Negril, Jamaica. You arrived skinny, pale and bald; you left so much stronger, with colour and more hair. It was transformational. You loved Ras Roddy outside on the West End Road, who sold street food – and more. You loved the Jamaican vibe, the plantain, the fish, the callaloo, jerk prawn and, of course, behind my back, the ganja.

On a future visit to another hotel on Negril Beach you visited Ras Roddy again. 'Johnnie, my man! Johnnie be goooood!' He gave you a chocolate brownie. 'Be careful. Share it with your friends, Johnnie!' A few days later, shortly before sunset when we'd have cocktails in the hot tub, I had a huge thirst for a cup of tea. 'We have that cake in the fridge!' I reminded him. How good it tasted – we ate it all, and soon followed it with a rum punch. The following twenty-four hours were some of the worst in my life. You found it funny that your straight, non-drug-taking wife had 'pulled a whitey', but you also had to take extreme care of me, as I became deeply paranoid and stoned for over a day. I hated every moment of it, but you were remarkably concerned and caring.

Winter sun became part of our annual agenda – it was the health tonic you needed to keep you strong. I would save through the year towards our holiday fund. Antigua, Saint Lucia, Grenada, Mauritius, Koh Samui and Australia were our winter destinations, as well as many more visits to Jamaica.

Australia was a destination that suited us both, as my brother Graham and your son Sam live in Sydney with their respective families. What joy we had with both of them. Their way of life was so enviable: sunshine, pools, decks, outdoor cooking, great beaches, fabulous food and wine. Byron Bay was a particular favourite. We loved the Indian Pacific train that took us from Perth across the enormous empty arid Nullarbor Plain (literally meaning 'no trees') to Sydney: three days of calm. We also had wine-maker friends Steve Webber and Leanne DeBortoli there, with whom we shared bottles of Pinot straight off the bottling plant followed by many of their repertoire of wines. They took us on tours of cellar doors in the Yarra Valley and the Mornington Peninsula, and shared good food, excellent wine and laughter like we've never known. Do you remember the plastic chicken you bought in a gift shop on Phillip Island? The evening became a hilarious celebration of Johnnie's Big Cock with their neighbours 'down the lane'. Steve and Leanne gave us lasting memo-ries, and gave me a belief that when I return, if I return, I want to be a winemaker.

We didn't just enjoy long haul, though. Short haul led us to the island of Paxos in Greece – an island that has given and given to us. Our first trip there was due to a photo of the small fishing village of Loggos on the Simpson Travel website. We loved its simplicity. Then I met someone at a local Dorset yoga class who had a house there. Frank Musker (coincidentally a songwriter for Chaka Khan, Aerosmith and Queen among others) and his wife, Rozzi, were people we were destined to meet. Time and again they would invite us to stay in their *spitáki*, so for years we loved going there in September. Thanks to Frank and Rozzi – known affectionately as 'the King and Queen of Paxos' – it was unbelievably social. It seems everyone went there: one night I sat next to the Rolling Stones' manager, and several other times we met up with leading rock musicians also on holiday there.

Island life is beautiful, small and simple; it gets under your skin. The other island we embraced was Tresco in the Isles of Scilly. You had always wanted to live by the sea, maybe because of all that time you spent on board the MV *Mi Amigo* when you were on Radio Caroline, and on Tresco we could own a week by the sea each year with their 'Islandshare' scheme. Our week in May in beautiful Seagrass overlooking the azure-blue sea towards St Martin's has been like a home from home and, happily, is very close to the gorgeous Ruin Beach Café, which to you meant black Americanos/croissant/pizza/wine/crab linguine and catch of the day. You loved that café so much, even more than the subtropical gardens, the beaches, the walks or the other islands. The Ruin was your ruin. That said, I did get you out for some walks before you became too limited. We loved to wander round to Gimble Porth and sit on a bench dedicated to Charles Baines. On it was the charming inscription, 'Let us sit together and watch for seals,' which we would do quietly, soaking up the beauty of the sea, land and rocky outcrops around us.

What you loved about me, and I about you, was that, while we adored an occasional taste of luxury, it didn't always have to be that way. We both enjoyed extremes – just not the in between. So when in 2008 you bought a white Auto-Trail

Cheyenne motorhome so that we could go on travel adventures together, I embraced the idea. You named her Martha, and we were the Van Dwellers – you, me and Darcey Dog. A motorhome, I discovered, can have many layouts. Martha had two bench sofas at the back with a table in between where we ate and played backgammon. At night you transformed this space into a double bed, the sofa cushions becoming mattresses. Martha had a tiny kitchenette complete with fridge, tiny sink, a loo and shower room. A wardrobe and head-height cupboards all round her gave storage for our clothes, books, DVDs and your vast selection of maps. She was the perfect size for two and a small dog. Plus, you got her an awning so that when we set up home in a campsite we could lay out a picnic table and chairs. It couldn't have been further away from a rock 'n' roll lifestyle.

How we loved getting Martha ready for trips. You would plan the journeys while I would organise food, bedding and backgammon. Our first trip was down the west coast of France. From Mont Saint-Michel to Santander in Spain. She was loaded with beautiful Emma Bridgewater colourful melamine plates, bowls and stripey cutlery and our two bicycles were attached at the back. Your bike to this day probably still sits in the Îsle de Ré bike shop, for it is there you fell for an electric bike, buying it for 1,000 euros and telling the man you'd be back to collect your own bike later. How you laughed as we drove out of town leaving it behind. You never were one for physical exertion, and you've always enjoyed an engine.

You had stayed in masses of campsites on biking trips, but as I had never camped, you were more than a little concerned about how I would deal with the shower blocks. How funny you found it to watch me waddling over to them with my towel and washbag. Fearing I would react badly, you gave me your assurance that I just had to say the word 'chateau' and we would be in one. I timed that word perfectly. When we arrived in Saint-Émilion the word slipped out of my mouth, we found an amazing chateau in the middle of the beautiful medieval town and got the final suite available. (Martha remained incognito in the town car park.) At reception they asked if we would like to dine there. You told them we'd think about it, and their eyebrows rose very discreetly. Only when we got to the room did I discover that it was at that time one of the top-fifty restaurants in the world. We took the last remaining table, and the food was magnificent.

With my fiftieth birthday under two years off, we decided to purchase the wine for my party there. Every spare crevice in Martha was stacked with bottles of fine Saint-Émilion Grand Cru, which still needed to be left a couple of years before drinking. By chance, the next night we met up with some friends who were also camping in France, and who were also bon vivants. Tom was then the general manager of Le Manoir aux Quat'Saisons – one of the finest hotels and restaurants in England. We parked up next to each other and after supper you suggested serving a rather fine wine. No one objected. Then Tom served a rather fine wine, and so it went on. What a night we had – £80 bottles being demolished in plastic camping wine glasses. We became so loud that other campers started to complain, and we were threatened with eviction from the site. Ha – two such upstanding Englishmen! The next day, with my future birthday wine stash seriously depleted, you drove away, quite illegally, given that I was still prostrate on the bed trying to sleep off my terrible hangover. Thank goodness for the onboard loo. I was kneeling in front of it as we made our way to Biarritz. It's a sad leftover of that night that I still cannot face Saint-Émilion wine, and at my fiftieth drank almost none of it, focusing on the champagne instead.

A Pembrokeshire coast trip allowed Darcey Dog to come with us. How she loved an adventure as much as you – new walks, beaches, sleeping tucked up next to me (where she thought you couldn't see her). How we loved the crashing seas and the characterful harbour villages. And on this trip we went one better: we towed my Fiat 500 behind us, so once we'd set up home on a campsite, we had freedom to travel.

Missing my production life so much, I did a few freelance producing jobs to keep my hand in, and you and Martha came on a couple of them. I'm not sure that the film crew could believe that Johnnie Walker was doing the craft services, but you were very good at it. Tea, coffee, snacks – you even got up at dawn to give the director and the cameraman a fry-up halfway up Snowdon on a Visit Wales commercial. In the Highlands of Scotland, where I was shooting a promo for the band Police Dog Hogan's track 'Fraserburgh Train', the budget was so small that Martha was the catering hub, production office, toilet facilities and wardrobe truck. Darcey came with us too on that job, and so beguiled was the director by her that she ended up being in it – running slow-mo across a mountain ridge, her black ears flying in the wind. Our girl immortalised! Your legs also featured, dressed in plus fours. Although we shot your whole body, you hit the cutting-room floor. Oh, the cruel rejection of an edit suite.

Martha was a fabulous asset to our lives. She was the perfect thing for festivals like Glastonbury, but the festival she's best remembered for was the Larmer Tree Festival on the Dorset–Wiltshire border, where not only did we entertain band Police Dog Hogan after their set, but later we managed to have an on-board disco with some friends, truly testing her suspension. It's ridiculous to love a vehicle, but we got everything down pat with her. Then one day, you went alone to a motorhome show in Birmingham, and thanks to your burning need to spend, and never being quite satisfied with what you've got, you traded her in. For £12,000 *more* you bought a smaller, vastly inferior grey Fiat van, and it's fair to say that I never forgave you. You tried to reason it by saying that Martha was too big for you to park these days. Realising that was unconvincing logic and that you'd made a stupid mistake, you tried to change your decision as soon as you got home, but dealers are bastards and you had to pay a huge premium if you wanted her back. It was the end of our camping days, for the grey thing was never liked by either Darcey or me. It was smaller, astonishingly uncomfortable and, frankly, we both missed the luxury and soul of dear Martha.

Our final holiday was in September 2023, in Greece, at a new hotel called the Mar-Bella Elix on the mainland. I was too nervous for us to stay on Paxos in case you fell ill. You were now struggling so badly with your lungs, just walking along the corridor to our room was hard for you; you had to stop several times to catch your breath and hold your chest. I lived in fear of you having a heart attack. You couldn't cope with the beach, for while there was a funicular to take us down to it – the very reason I chose the hotel – there were then over twenty steps to go right down to the beach, and you just couldn't do it. You remained by the pool, and each morning I would pop down alone for my daily sea swim.

The irony of the location was that the hotel looked out directly onto Paxos. Every day my heart ached to be on our special island where we had friends, cafés and beaches we loved, and the boats to Antipaxos, the small island just off Paxos, which we adored visiting. It got too much for me. I went to ask the hotel tour desk how we could pop over for the day to see friends for coffee. The only option was the weekly tourist boat trip to Paxos, which stopped in the main town of Gaios for forty-five minutes. It cost 240 euros for both of us. There was no choice. I booked it and we were met at the harbour by Frank and Rozzi, plus our other island friends James and Catherine. Frank looked at me sipping my cappuccino and just said, 'You are Paxos people.' How I knew it. The boat trip went on to Antipaxos and into the caves on the west of the island, and because you love boats it was a good day, even though you weren't fit enough to jump into the sea for a swim with me. Back at the hotel the girl at the tour desk asked if we'd seen our friends OK. I said we had. 'Good, because that was the most expensive coffee you'll ever have.' She wasn't wrong, but how happy I was that you got to see our beloved Greek island just one more time.

The thought of you not being my travelling companion one day fills me with huge sadness. We really have been brilliant together, and honestly, they have been our best times.

OUR TEN BEST ADVENTURES

Tensing Pen, Negril, Jamaica – our first time to the Caribbean and where you truly healed from your cancer treatment.

Venice – we went three times in November or March. You loved the boat taxi from the airport to the hotel as you felt like James Bond. The best was when we returned on the Orient Express.

La Residencia in Deià – our 'not the honeymoon' where you say you truly fell in love with me.

Taking Martha the Motorhome on her inaugural trip down the west coast of France, bringing back St-Émilion wine and an early electric bike.

Taking the Indian Pacific train across Australia from Perth to Sydney.

Visiting Steve and Leanne Webber of De Bortoli Wines on the Mornington Peninsula. When you mix a magical setting with great hosts, fine wine, amazing food, hilarious company and visits to cellar doors at niche vineyards, life doesn't get much better.

All our holidays on Paxos.

The first time I took you to Tresco. You loved it, as I knew you would. Having always wanted a house by the sea, you could fulfil that dream by getting an Islandshare house there – a beautiful coastal pad just for one week of the year.

Your niece Trudi's wedding to Todd in Vancouver, which we followed with a drive to the stunning Emerald Lake, and a train ride from Vancouver to Seattle.

The Great Wall of China. Truly extraordinary to be taken along the wild wall section by the expert William Lindesay. After one week of utterly basic living we took our Carers UK fundraising group of friends to the Chinese Embassy in Beijing to have the poshest tea surrounded by fine art, thanks to our friend Dame Barbara Woodward who was then the UK's Ambassador to China.

NOW

IF I WERE A RICH MAN

'I wish we were rich.' Where did that come from? Money has a loud voice, but it doesn't have soul. You have soul, Johnnie Walker – that's far more important. Besides, what can you possibly do with money now? (Except pay for some carers so I can have time out. I know they're expensive.)

You've just been texting with John Illsley (of Dire Straits), who told you about the party they have just thrown in a big marquee in the garden of their spectacular home. I guess we would have been there in healthier times. You start imagining how amazing it would have been, with wonderful guests, catering and decoration. You don't mention music, but I can only assume that was pretty good too.

You and money were never destined to go together. It was not in your stars. I know it's galling that because you are a big radio name people assume you are wealthy, but they don't realise that radio really is the poor relation of the BBC. 'I'm not a star like Wogan and Graham Norton,' you always said. You are right; you are just a jock and have always been paid as such. If you wanted to be rich, you would have taken that offer from Smooth Radio all those years ago, or done a Ken Bruce and gone to Greatest Hits, but we both know that the BBC is your home. You get fabulous production, you've always enjoyed great guests, you get incredible support – especially now – and you are the grandfather of the Radio 2 family. Plus, there are no ads.

When we met you were in a rented flat and you had huge debts due to the legal fees of fighting the *News of the World* sting. And let's face it, you are profligate with money. My accountant, GT, became *our* accountant. 'Walker pisses money up against the wall,' was his quickly formed, astute observation. Buying has been one of your addictions, but look where you are now? In a house that you like and I still shop at Waitrose. Just. I remind you how lucky we are. How we have everything we need. How we are better off than most. I guess it's just that we have spent quite a bit of time with people far richer than ourselves and you compare yourself with them. We are so often the poor guests who keep our heads held high because you are Johnnie Walker. I am proud of that and what you have achieved. I know you are too, but you seem bemused as to why it hasn't resulted in a healthier bank balance.

This desire of yours to be rich goes back a long way. 'Why aren't you wealthy like Noel Edmonds?' your mother would goad you when you were at Radio 1 in the 1970s. I see that went deep. You saw failure in her eyes, as she was just judging you by financial success. I remind you, yet again, that what you have now – love, respect and a Radio 2 show

– still, at the age of seventy-nine, is way beyond what Noel Edmonds could dream of having. I'm sure he'd cash in every helicopter he's ever owned to be in the position you are now. Do not measure yourself in financial terms. Look at your longevity and the legacy you will leave. As I always tell you, you should be so proud, because the love for you will live on. I promise. You only half hear this.

It is a credit to your ego that you have no idea just how important you are and have been in radio, to thousands of listeners, but you have been. You have a very special voice that touches souls – I'd almost say your voice heals. And when you go you will be irreplaceable. When you look down on your life from above that is what you will see, and you will realise that it was a life well lived (with a few blips). There is no money in heaven. Indeed, the rich have a hard time getting in according to the Bible. You are rich, Johnnie, just not in the obvious bank-balance way – and you cannot take that with you. You are rich in love from your listeners. Just look at the emails and cards that flow in day after day telling you how great you are and how missed you will be. That love you most certainly will take with you. It is the greatest currency.

It's 26 June 2024, my half-birthday, which as a child I always celebrated because Boxing Day is arguably the worst day of the year for an actual birthday. It remains special to me to this day, although I don't shout about it. You mark it – bless you. I wake at our little London flat in Primrose Hill

– the one that Darcey Dog selected for us. As a puppy she couldn't cope with the pavements near the BBC so a walk on Primrose Hill had her tail wagging furiously. We saw this flat with her and, while we were looking at the bedroom, she was busy taking a house plant out of its pot in the sitting room, spreading soil all over the cream carpet. She literally marked the place – so we swapped the flat near the BBC for this one. I came up last night to see my niece Brigitte, who has flown in from Sydney with her husband and girls. It is so good to see them, to sit in the Riding House Café drinking cocktails and red wine, catching up after five years when we have lost her amazing mother, Kim, and two of my brothers, Simon and Emlyn. I guess you are next.

I sleep so well in Primrose Hill. It is much quieter these days; since Covid no one goes out till the small hours. It's certainly quieter than the middle of nowhere where we live – no cockerels, cows or magpies fighting. It is bliss! I feel as if I have come on holiday. Just one night away from our open prison of a home is such a relief – as good as going to a Caribbean island. I feel so free. I see the matinee of *A View from the Bridge* with Dominic West; it's excellent. The audience love it, and I am part of something bigger than being your carer. I am carried completely by Arthur Miller's gripping story. I even find an actor for my film – a birthday present to myself. Our friends Rodney and Mariana have got you covered during the day, and your daughter Beth stays with you overnight. Thank you to them for this twenty-four hours of freedom.

I return home on a crowded, hot train. I collect wood-fired pizzas from the Grosvenor Arms and rush them back to you, waiting for me with a card, flowers and a new tennis skirt. Separation is so healthy. I babble with excitement, tell you the plot of the play, drink red wine, eat too much pizza. I am just so happy. It's one of my best ever half-birthdays. And doubtless my last one with you. You are genuinely pleased to see me sparkle again. It's been too long.

You soon have something important to discuss with me, though. I pretty much know what is coming. I can see it hasn't worked for you – its ability to move up and down does nothing for you; it brings you no comfort; the duvet falls off every night: you hate the mattress. You don't have enough space to lay out your iPad and phone. You look too big for it. So yes, I will move the hospital bed out and bring back in your much-loved four-foot divan bed from where it sits, lonely, in the garage. Thank heavens I didn't give it away. You just have to wait until I can get some help. It was quite an undertaking doing the swap in the first place.

I move you and your concentrator to my room. I thought you'd slept in this bed for the last time, but here you are, back in the marital bed! Mariana and I strip the offending NHS bed and then realise we can't even get it through the door. It is so heavy we can't possibly lift it. I call the district nurse's office and they say I mustn't attempt to disassemble it. You stay in my bed all day, sleeping like a baby, possibly relieved to be on a beautiful mattress again. You stay there for the night but insist on using your bathroom. I go in the guest room but continue to use my en-suite bathroom. I lie in bed with criss-cross images in my head. It's all wrong. The feng shui is not working. Neither of us sleep well, both discombobulated by the wrongness of the set-up.

Sarah, who had been our cleaner and support mechanism for so many years of our marriage before she retired, is coming to see us. We agree that if anyone can sort this, Sarah can. Especially if we ask our neighbour John to help out. He's a helicopter pilot; he can do anything. Together they work out how to take the bed apart. I don't care if we shouldn't. I just want you to be back in the safe haven of your room. They carry it to the garage and bring back your beloved bed. I never thought Sarah would be making up a bed for us again, but in she went, duvet and cover in hand, hospital corners for the bottom sheet. You are so happy in that bed I can't get you out of it until suppertime.

'What's on the menu tonight?' you ask at about 6 p.m., as you do each evening as you decide whether to have a G&T, a glass of wine or just water with your bowl of Kettle crisps.

'Friday night is Dirty Burger Night.' You are delighted. Dirty Burger Night happens as a treat about once a month. For you, it's a Linda McCartney vegetarian one; for me, it's Waitrose rose veal. You always ask, 'Why is it a "dirty" burger?' and I always tell you that it's because Suzi Perry calls it that, as do many. We had been at a carers' awards do, and we'd invited a few names to sit at our table – Michael Ball, Tony Blackburn, Anneka Rice and Suzi Perry. Once all the wonderful carers had been acknowledged for their self-less work, and the dinner had been cleared, you and Suzi still had a glint in your eye. Loving to be led astray, you readily agreed when she suggested we go on for a drink. We went on for several in the end, and at some point in the early hours Suzi announced that we needed a dirty burger. She knew the bar of a hotel near Park Lane. I am always impressed by people who know where to go at any time of the day or night to eat or drink. I was also impressed that she didn't eat her bun – but then she works on TV, and I don't; I needed the blotting paper. It was the first and last time that we took a cab back home as the sun was coming up. We giggled at the naughtiness of it, and fell into bed for a long, deep sleep.

Tonight's effort isn't my best dirty burger ever – the beef tomato was sliced a bit too thick, and I added a lettuce leaf too many – and you struggle to eat yours. But then you have started to mention more and more how hard it is to eat and breathe. You go very slowly. You remove most of the salad.

As a dinner conversation you talk about IPF symptoms towards the end of life. Not the best meal-time discussion, but it's the one time of the day when we really look into each other's eyes. You've been doing more research, and hearing from listeners who have lost a family member to it. It has always been a risk that you would pick up an infec-tion and drop like a stone, but you've got through the winter. (You seem to be impervious to infections. You are the only person I know who never got Covid.) So it seems that the slowing down and sleeping more is your natural path to the end. That said, after supper you say that you're bored of this now. 'Dirty burgers?' I ask. No, the fighting to breathe and everything being such an almighty effort. It is Friday, 28 June. I wonder if your soul will hear you, for I feel you will determine when you go. What is money when life has actually become too much effort to live? Some things money cannot buy, and one of those is health.

LOVE ME, LOVE MY DOG

If I were to give thanks for just one thing in our marriage, it would be Darcey Dog. It cannot be understated just what a special creature she was. Unable as we were to have children together, she was our surrogate child. You, me and her: that was our family.

You initiated her arrival, hearing about a litter of working cocker spaniels in the New Forest. We'd already had one working cocker – dear Fergus – who, while we loved him hugely, was a tad too wild for us as you recovered from cancer. Fergus was adopted by Madonna's estate manager, Willy. As Martin Shankleman, your former business correspondent on *Drivetime*, observed, 'Fergus just used you, Johnnie, to get up the showbiz ladder.' I believe that to this day Guy Ritchie still has Fergus's offspring at Ashcombe.

When we met Darcey's litter the extrovert ones bounded over to me, but the quiet, rather insecure and bullied runt came and sat at your feet. She looked up at you with her pleading eyes. 'Hello,' you said, picking her up. Darcey chose you. She recognised something in you, and weeks later home she came. Her confidence grew, and living as we did then in the Granary, on the edge of a farm with a pheasant shoot, she had a great youth chasing pheasants and deer. How that girl could run.

At puppy class we realised she pretty much disliked most other dogs, but she adored humans – she could get her way with them. Our mad theory was always that she was Lady Diana reincarnated, because she shared those same eyes looking up pleadingly from under her fringe. Plus, she truly was the people's pooch. She was loved wherever she went, which sometimes included your interviews in London. She was a hit with Patti Smith and met more rockstars than I ever did.

Her traits were delightful. When she was excited she'd cock her body round in a curve, wagging that docked tail with vigour, and she tried to talk. Of course, she could bark, but she had more in her vocabulary. She really tried to convey her emotions with a call-cum-squeal that revealed her mood. There was intonation in her voice, and we would stand before her, asking, 'What are you saying, Darcey?' and she'd honestly appreciate our efforts to understand. She considered herself just as human as us.

She adapted between her Dorset and Primrose Hill life with delight. She loved the contrast: pheasants in the country; squirrels in London. She didn't care what she chased. She never caught anything, but oh, the challenge of trying. Her stumpy tail would wag furiously as she hysterically squealed with excitement. That dog loved life, loved people, loved us. She also loved to be good. Her favourite compliment was, 'You're such a good girl, Darcey.' She really appreciated that acknowledgement. She was a wonderful example to us all, and her spirit touched all who she met. As such, she had a wonderful social life, went for walks with many of her human friends and knew more people in Shaftesbury than we ever did.

She only ever went to a kennel for two nights of her life. There were too many people offering to have her to stay. Her first godmother was Sarah, our right-hand woman for many years, and then when we moved to Shaftesbury her new godparents were our friends Jonathan and Claire. It didn't matter what mischief she got up to, they all adored her. She could do no wrong, just entertain.

She was going blind and deaf and becoming arthritic by the time she was fourteen, but that didn't stop her having the best week of her life when we took her to Tresco in November on a 'doggie break' – the only occasion Tresco allows people to bring their dogs to the island. After the plane and boat ride, she knew when she got there that the place was special. She ran around ecstatically – it was quite extraordinary how she reacted. Finally, she was joining us in one of our favourite places and it was as if she knew that. She and I walked every inch of the island's paths and beaches together. She didn't want to leave, but whoever does?

Four months later in 2022 was Storm Eunice. As I explained to Darcey, the BBC said we weren't to go out walking because of the danger. It was the only day of her life this had happened, and it was not well received. Later that night, after she'd happily polished off the remains of your supper, we had a power cut. We decided to go to bed early, so you let her out for her final pee. What you didn't tell me was that she'd turned right and not left into the fenced in part of the garden. After a while I commented that she'd been a long time. We both took turns looking in the garden with a torch, but she wasn't there. She had clearly taken herself off for a hooley. We called our neighbours in case she was in their gardens. Mark across the drive from us got out his truck, and in the pitch black we went searching the local roads. There was no sign of her. It was a bitterly cold night. Back home, empty-handed, I put up a post on the Nextdoor app. During her life she'd torn off on quite a few occasions, but she was always found. This time I had a very different feeling in the pit of my stomach.

Even though I felt it was hopeless I was up early the next morning scouring fields. So were many people in the area. Our home became Rescue HQ, with people descending on us and conducting their own search parties or using drones. I would stop strangers to ask them to look out for her, only to discover that they were already out looking for her. Hundreds of people searched for that little dog.

After three days my only way to deal with it was to sit in bed and write. I never wanted to forget a single detail of her last precious day:

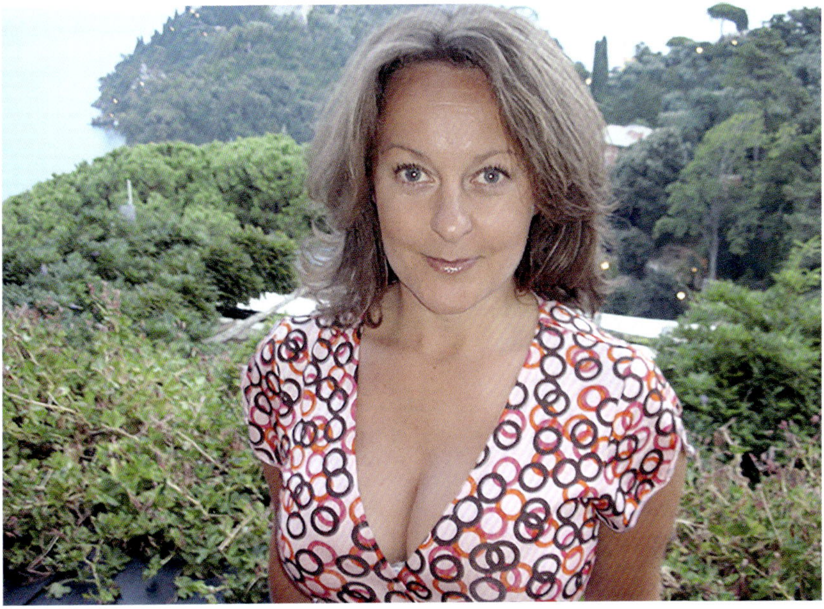

At the Hotel Splendido, September 2003. Oh what a night!

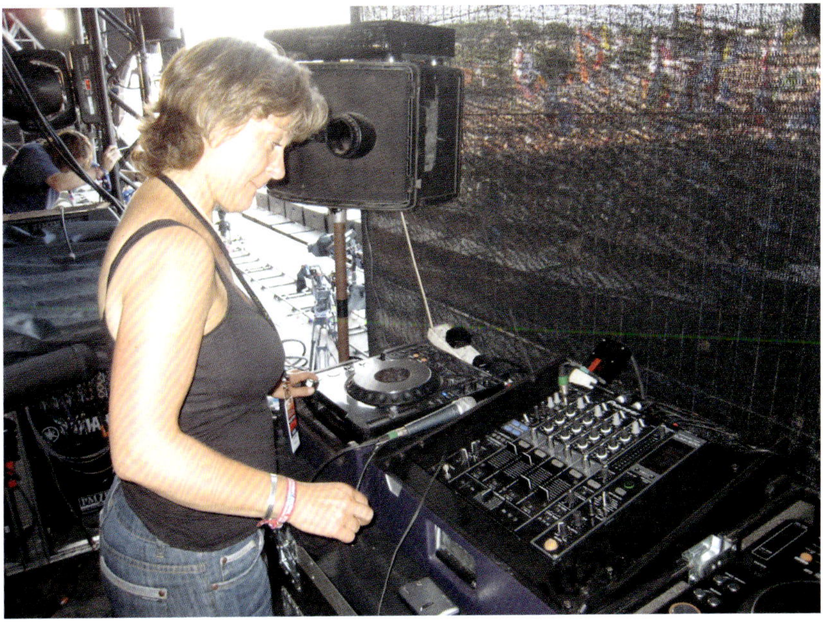

My moment of megalomania – DJ'ing on the Pyramid Stage at Glastonbury, 2009.

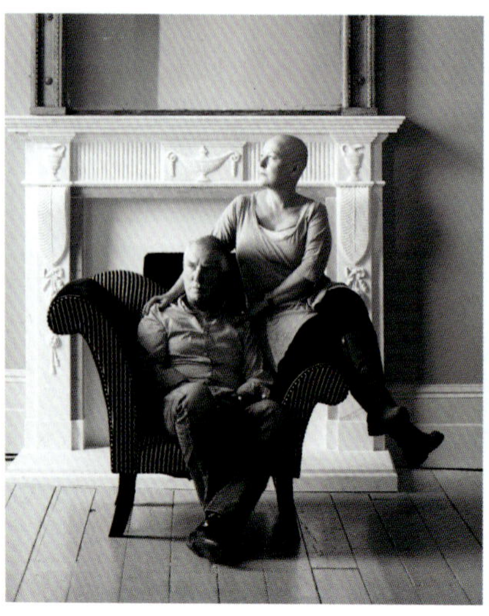

Me and Johnnie during my chemo months, 2014.

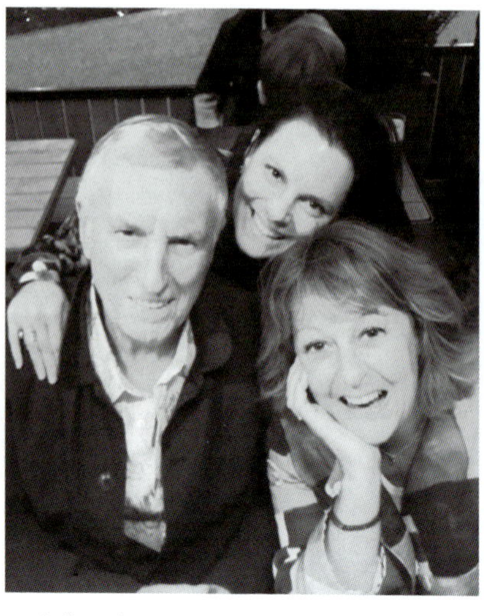

A full circle moment with our friend Carly Cook – she edited Johnnie's biography and is now my agent.

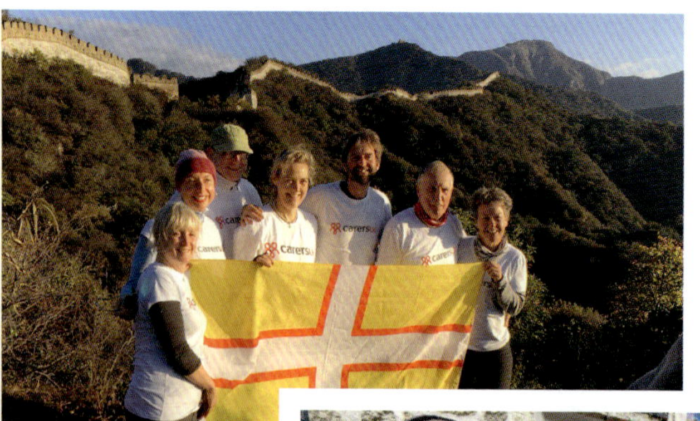

Fundraising with our Dorset friends for Carers UK. Sunrise on the Great Wall of China, October 2017.

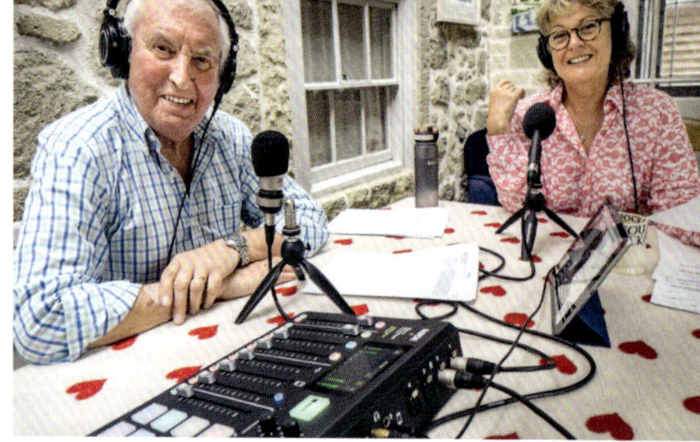

Recording *Sounds of the 70s* together from home during lockdown one.

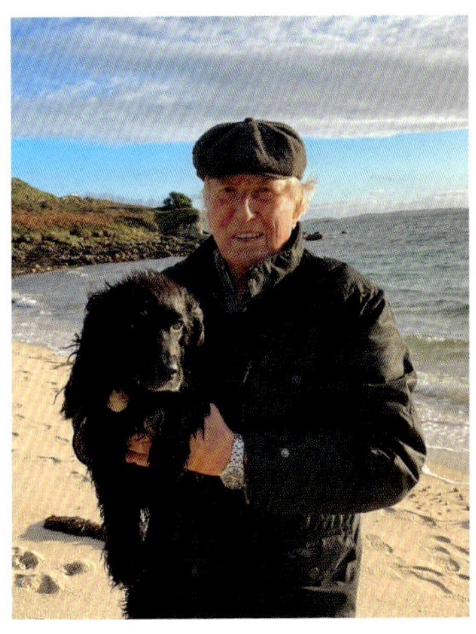

Darcey's doggy holiday on Tresco, November 2021. Her finest week.

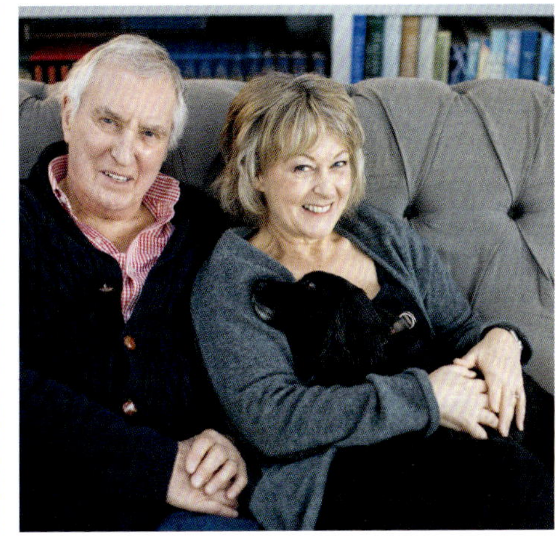

Our last photo with Darcey in 2021. I may be holding her but it's Johnnie who she looks up to with adoration.

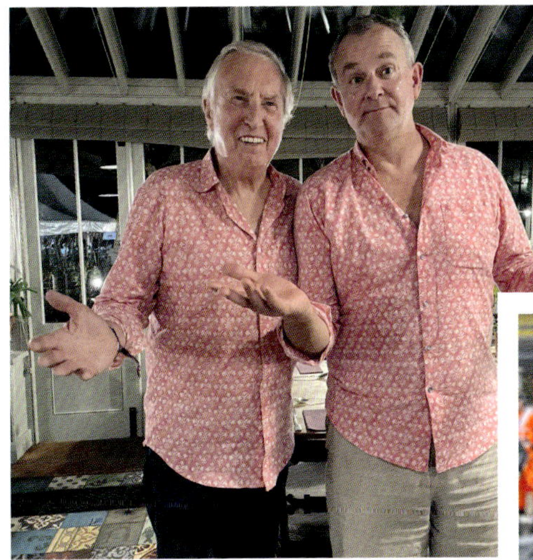

ABOVE: What are the chances? Johnnie and Hugh Bonneville turn up to The Pig Hotel Smoked & Uncut festival in the same shirt.

RIGHT: The F1 Gridwalk at Silverstone, July 2021. It was THE place to be in the world at that moment and a true privilege.

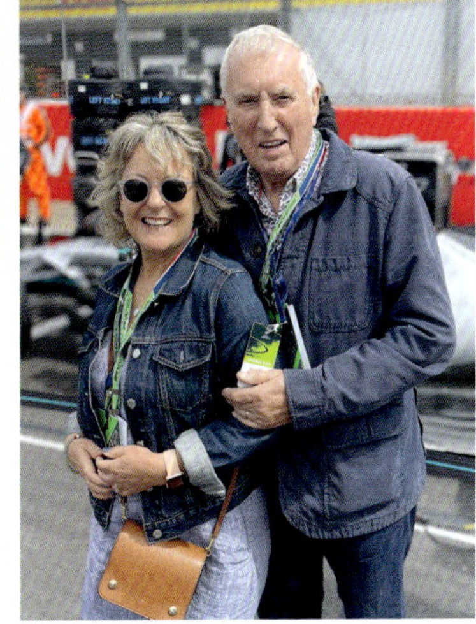

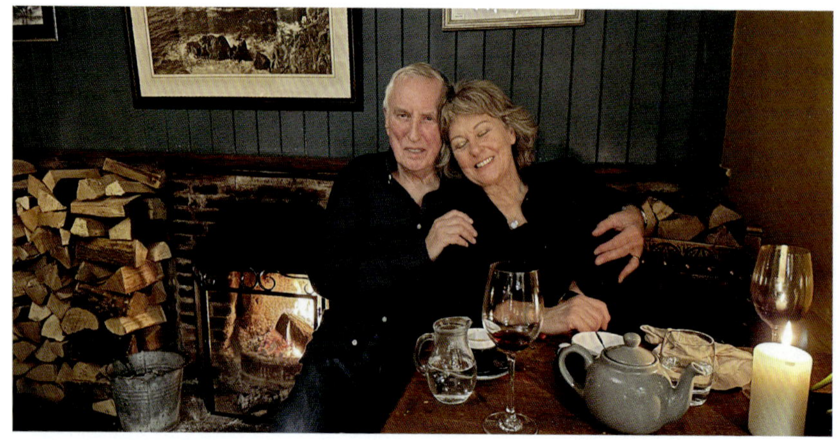

Our 20th Wedding Anniversary at The Gurnard's Head, Cornwall, December 2022. The last time Johnnie was strutting. His downfall started the next day when he fell out of a helicopter.

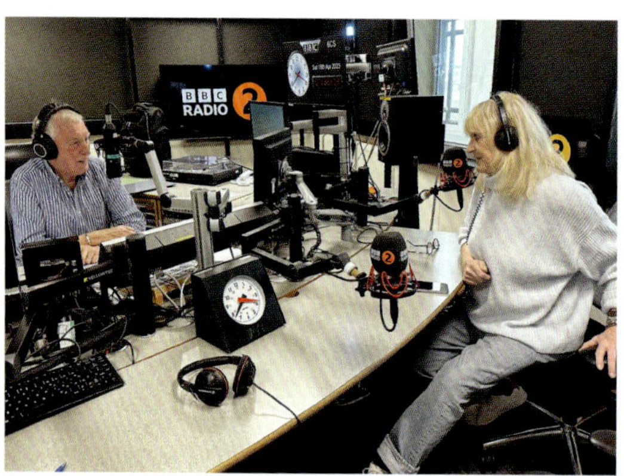

Delighted to see his old 'bounce' Sally Traffic while standing in on *Sounds of the 60s*, April 2023.

The mystery of 'Jakemansgate' is solved. Johnnie repentant with Michael Ball outside Wogan House.

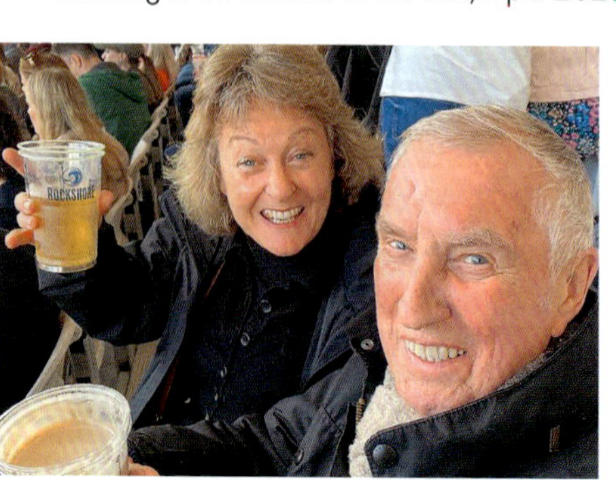

LEFT: Last gig together . . . Bruce Springsteen at the RDS in Dublin, May 2023.

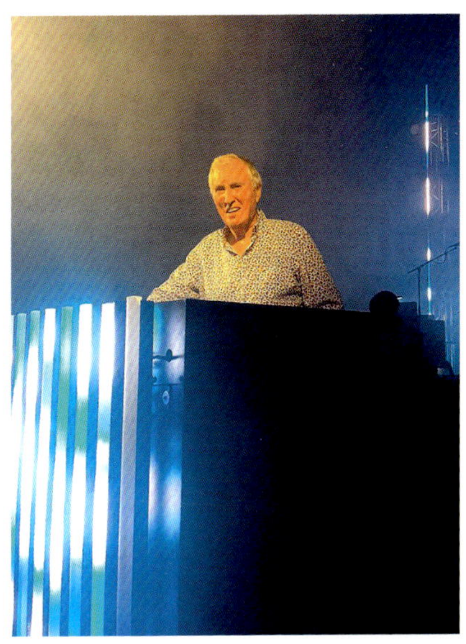

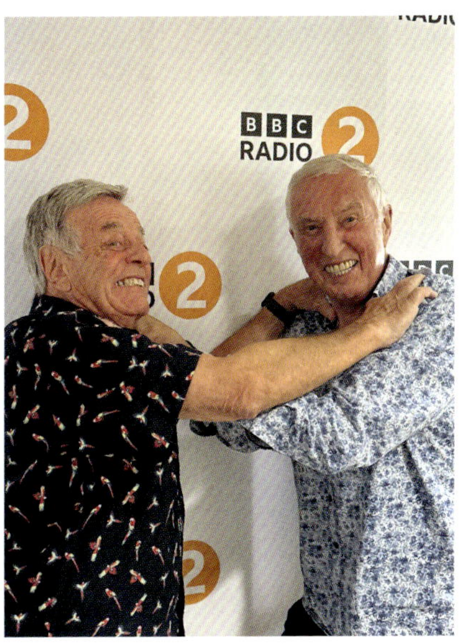

DJ'ing at Versailles Palace, July 2023, in his final public appearance.

Johnnie and Tony Blackburn fighting it out at Radio 2 after recording 'Clash of The Pirates', 2023.

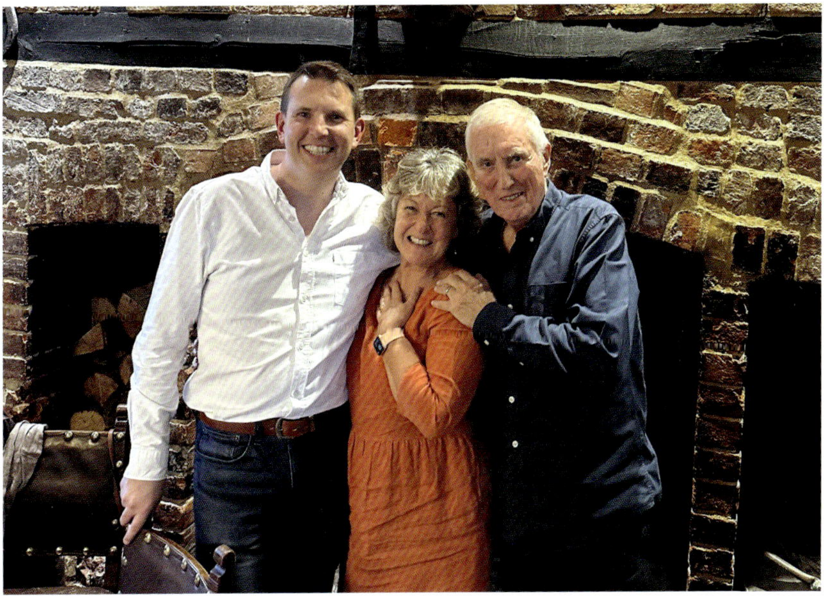

Johnnie's son, Sam, visits from Australia, November 2023. Sunday lunch at The Grosvenor Arms, Hindon.

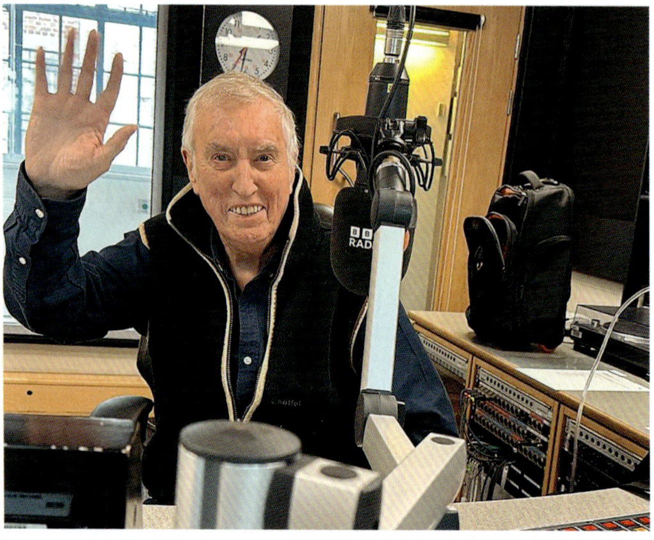

Johnnie's final live show at Radio 2, New Year's Eve 2023.

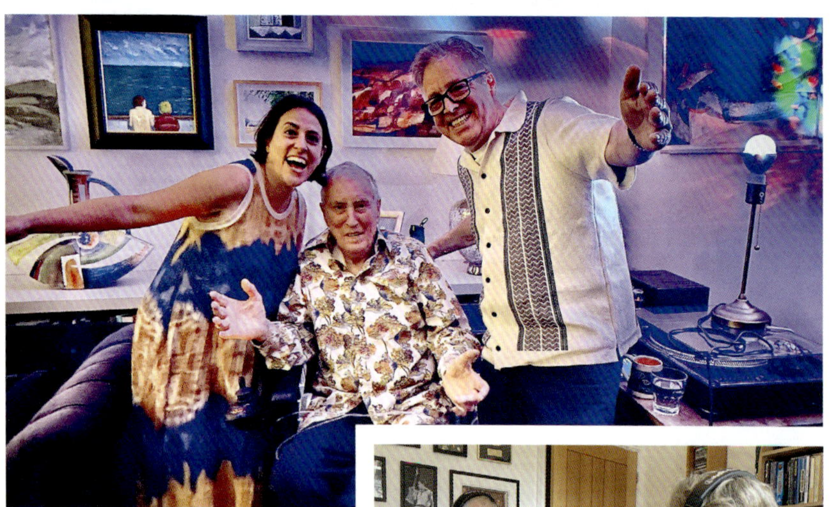

ABOVE: Kitchen Disco, August 2024, with Johnnie's boss Helen Thomas and fellow DJ Mark Goodier.

RIGHT: Johnnie and me recording his last *Sounds of the 70s* show in his den at home, October 2024.

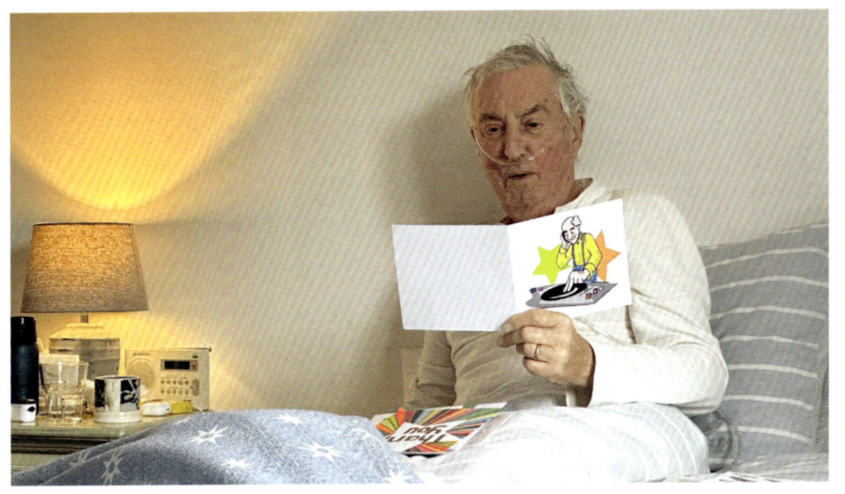

ABOVE: Retired with time to read all the many 'thank you' cards he was sent.

ABOVE: The day Michael and Emily Eavis came for tea – in the drive.

RIGHT: A morning fag and Irish coffee in the usual attire, with the post on his lap, December 2024.

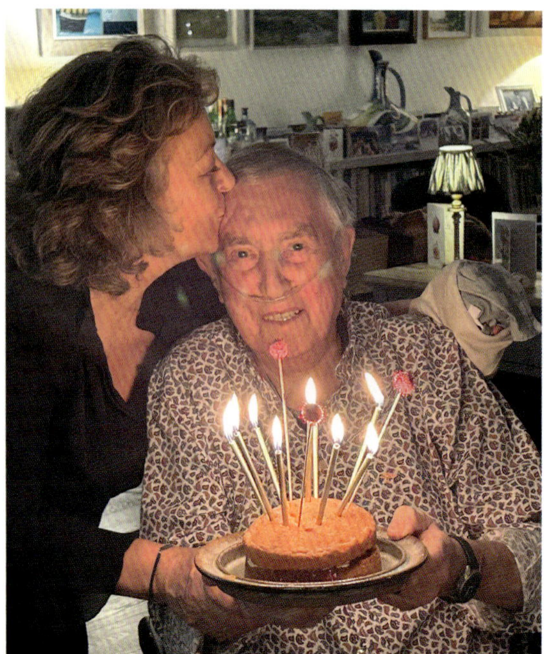

My 64th birthday, December 2024. But whose cake is it? The last ever photo of Johnnie taken by our friend, Jane Treays. He died five days later.

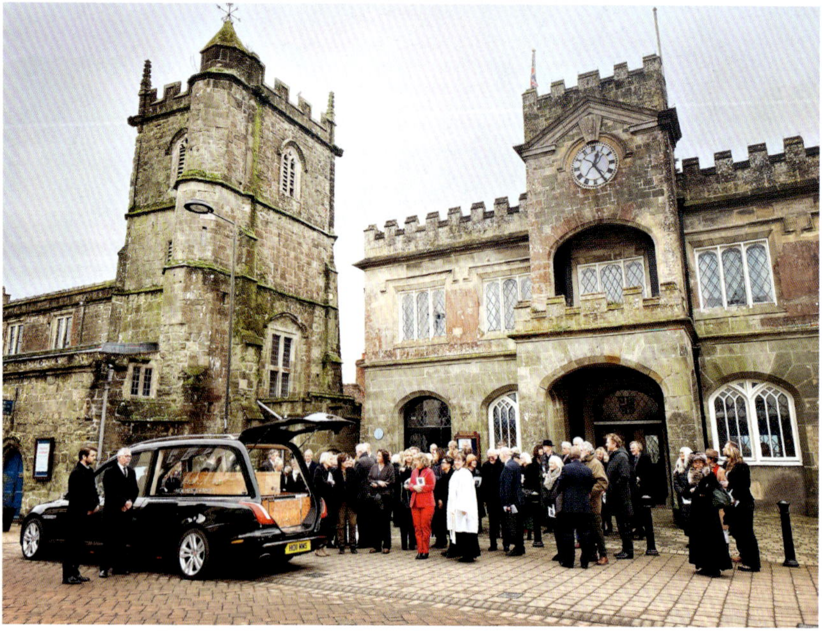

Outside Johnnie's funeral at St Peters Church, Shaftesbury, January 2025. He was taken away with 'Born to Run' blaring from the hearse.

Is Celeriac Poisonous for Dogs? Darcey's Final Day.

I sat on the stool by the grey sofa watching her sleep. She looked so content, her legs stretched out, her head comfortably resting on two blue linen cushions. As if she'd finally mastered human pillow habits. She stood up and wagged her stump of a tail, shoving her nose close to mine. On this day she was particularly happy and bouncy. She tore around the kitchen, skidding on the wooden floor and crashing into chairs. I drew the long grey linen curtains to open the bifold door to the garden. Out she tore. Throwing herself on the lawn and arching her back as she rolled in this blissful daily wake-up manoeuvre, her tail wagging throughout. She returned, leaping back across the threshold of the door, bringing in the smallest smudge of mud across her head.

By lunchtime Storm Eunice had kicked off. Our bins had all gone flying, recycling spreading itself across the lawn and newspapers splatting against our fence before crossing to our neighbour's garden and then into the field beyond. As Johnnie tried to grab what he could, Darcey joined him, cantering around, her head towards the considerable wind, her ears flying back and up.

This storm had changed the daily pattern. I lay back on the grey sofa against the two blue linen cushions with a post-yoga cup of tea. Such novelty appealed to Darcey, who came up for a cuddle. I pointed out that the mud was still on her topknot and she needed a bath. This fell on unwilling ears, and she sloped off in case I meant 'now'.

It was a simple supper for the humans that evening. Sea bass, spinach and celeriac purée. The latter was remarkably sharp. Making it with zero-fat quark did it no favours. Johnnie didn't finish his. Darcey was in luck. Sea bass skin, and his rejected celeriac, was going spare. She wolfed it all down.

The power cut happened soon after 9 p.m. There was nothing to do but go to bed. It was customary for her to spend about five minutes outside at night, having a good sniff around all the corners of the garden. But when we looked outside she was nowhere. We searched the local roads, but went to bed feeling sick.

The next morning I was up early searching the cow shed up the lane, going to speak to neighbours and walking her favourite fields. For two days stacks of friends and people we've never met were out, many taking dogs.

At some point Johnnie joked, 'I think it was your celeriac purée.' And tonight, three days since she left us, I found myself googling 'Is celeriac poisonous for dogs?' I am happy to discover it is not and is full of nutrients.

I'm glad she had a little extra in her tummy when she left. I hope it kept her warm on what was a blisteringly cold night. I hope desperately that she departed this world in a moment of euphoria, giddy on the wildness of the night. She has been such a very special dog her entire life, bringing joy and love to so many, that she deserved nothing less. For me, my heart has to hold on to that image because any thought of her suffering is too heart-breaking to bear.

I shall never forget Darcey. I shall never forget Storm Eunice. I shall always blame the power cut. And I will never eat celeriac again.
22/2/22

I remember your phone call as I was driving back from town five days after she'd gone. 'Where are you, Duch?' You had never, ever called me to ask where I was, so I knew it was about Darcey. As I got out of the car I said, 'She's home, isn't she?' You nodded, told me she was in the garden. Mark, our neighbour, was a local farmer and had found her and brought her back. I just wasn't expecting to see her little body wrapped tightly in a blue blanket. I could see the rigid shape of her frame, her legs, her nose. I let out a scream so deep that I had no idea I was capable of such a sound. It was my primal scream. You had been in the middle of recording your *Sounds of the 70s* show when she was brought back. You had to record the second half of the show having just discovered that our 'daughter' had drowned in a local pond on what had been the coldest night of the year.

I called Jonathan and Claire. Within minutes they were round with Jake, their son. The two men dug Darcey's grave and, after both you and Jonathan had bravely groomed her, you wrapped her up once more and laid her in it. All we could do was hold each other in our grief.

My wonderful dog-loving editor Helen Stiles at *Dorset Magazine* read my tribute to Darcey and said that not only could it be my next month's column but that she'd give me three pages. She paid Darcey the highest compliment, saying she'd have put the photo of her smiling on Tresco on the cover of the magazine if it had been taken in Dorset.

Weeks later we had a funeral for her. About thirty of her friends, godparents and family attended. Even my mother came. You gave a brief eulogy, and our friend and old mucker, the psychic, Tarot-reading Big Pete, recited a poem he had written for her, with us all gathered around. Afterwards we had lunch. It was a beautiful day and send-off to the most amazing dog anyone there had ever known.

Darcey chose you. And while I did all the walking and feeding and scheduling of her diary (yes, she had a diary!), she looked up to you as the master of our pack. In the last photo of the three of us together she lies across me, but looks up to you with such devotion and love. There is no doubt that for both of us the first encounter we both look forward to in heaven is with Darcey Dog, her black body cocking round in a curve, her stumpy tail wagging and her delightful doggy voice welcoming us.

Friends asked about getting another dog, but how could we replace such a special creature? Not only would it feel disloyal, but almost certainly it would be a disappointment after the one and only Darcey Walker. She was sent to us by divine providence, and one day maybe another will be sent to me. If so, I think it will be a miniature sausage dog … called Sizzle.

THEY SHOOT HORSES, DON'T THEY?

It's 1 July 2024, six months since your health crashed and both our lives changed. Last night I had an unusual dream for me – it was incredibly clear. I was on a train pulling into Tisbury station and there you were in your beautiful cord jacket you bought in Venice (now sold on Vinted). You were tall, strong, handsome – and you were standing. You have always loved meeting me at the station – the joy of reconnection and being one again. It was so beautiful to see you like that. Whoever knew that your husband standing on a train platform could be a thing of such profound joy. We learn too late, don't we?

Six months in: a point I never imagined you would make, but there you are, soul intact, *Rock Show* recorded for today and waiting to watch your crush Emma Raducanu play at Wimbledon. While you seem perfectly fine given your basic level of existence, I have never felt so deeply and profoundly exhausted. I've a column to finish for *Dorset Magazine* and for the first time ever, I have no energy or inspiration to write it. A first-time writer's block. I put it down to fatigue.

I spoke with an old friend, Karin, earlier. We shared a room when we both worked in Paris in 1980. She has taken a spiritual and coaching route through life. I tell her my deep-rooted fear that you will outlive me as I am going to get overcome with exhaustion and fall ill. She impresses upon me that I must change my thinking. She is a great believer in the 'law of attraction', whereby if you think a thing too much it will become reality. I must change my mindset. But you are so sodding strong and I see no sign of you letting go. 'I've carried him and his life for twenty-two years. I don't know how much longer I can go on,' I tell her. She understands. All my friendship group know I keep our show on the road. How I have ever since we got married. Today I am longing to know when it can be a solo show. Not because I don't love you – I do so deeply and will miss you incredibly – but I just want to curl up in a ball and sleep for days without letting you down. I want to be off the hook, to go to the cinema and be free to stay out all day. Indeed, I really want to go and see Kevin Costner's *Horizon* at the Everyman in Salisbury tomorrow, but I've not found the right moment to tell you, for I know that it will fill me with guilt. Carer's guilt. How long will this go on? Will six months become twelve? You're going to finish me off if we're not careful.

Another show day. It's Wednesday, so today is *Sounds of the 70s*. Every pre-recorded show is checked by someone in management before it airs. You say you've never been so censored in what you can say or play as a result. You love telling people that you cannot play 'Hong Kong Garden' or the Goons' 'The Ying Tong Song' because they are deemed racist. Pre-records have kept your career going, but I know it frustrates you. If a guest ever mentions having a spliff or any drugs in the Seventies, it is cut out before it airs. Only last week, when you interviewed music PR Alan Edwards, the story about him being backstage in someone's dressing room with a Hells Angel who got him to play Russian Roulette with a loaded pistol was removed. It's always the best stories that are taken out. How you love a live interview and show – no one can censor you then. You can just apologise.

I take you your black coffee and Berocca Boost as usual. I turn your oxygen down to Level 5 so the mic doesn't pick up the sound. You and Liz talk about the show, and then I hear your voice do a total gear change as you start to record. How do you do it? You project, you sound strong, you are humorous. I tell you, your listeners don't know how lucky they are. They get the very best of you – the last remaining strands of the old Johnnie. You showman, you. Doctor Showbiz doing his bit.

I'm left with an exhausted husk who I put to bed early after I've undressed him. Tonight, you cry at bedtime. We're side by side on your bed as you hold my arm. 'I'm sorry I'm going to leave you,' you sob. You talk about what a hard time we have been put through during our marriage – the illnesses, the challenges. How strong we have had to be to keep going, how incredible it is that we have. Especially me. You apologise that you have let me down at times, that you have not loved me with the strength and goodness with which I have loved you. You tell me that my pure heart has taught you so much. Honestly, darl, I may be as loyal as they come, but I'm really not *that* special a person, yet you truly believe I am, and I love that about you. You make me feel special, though really I'm just well brought up by two very moral, good, loving, intelligent human beings. I was taught to put others before myself. To recognise those worse off than me, and not to envy those who have it better. To you, that makes me a saint.

To be honest, I've cried today too, but only because I am so depleted of energy. It frightens me when I am like this, as I know from experience that it means my immune system is getting low. I am known for being positive – which of course I am still in public, but even that is getting more taxing.

Johnnie, I miss our life together so very much. You have been my playmate for almost twenty-three years; now you are my charge who I must care for. I know I am lucky to have this transitional time with you, but honestly, the grieving has not only started already; it has well and truly taken hold.

I'm slightly concerned that my final words to you will be, 'I'm bloody knackered.'

I notice how much you tell me you love me when I say goodnight. When I walked into my room tonight you texted me too, just for good measure: 'Tiggy, I love you SO much.' Are you trying to tell me something? You will be there in the morning, won't you? Am I reading too much into a text because a deeply hidden part of my subconscious is hoping it is nearly over?

As you know, I am the Queen of the Diary. I adore scheduling – an important production skill – and have always spent hours on it so that our life flows as well and efficiently as it possibly can. It started when Terry Wogan was alive and you filled in for three months of his *Radio 2 Breakfast Show* each year. That was the backbone of our year's planning. Everything else, such as holidays and events, would come on the back of Terry and Helen's plans. Since then, it has been based around your shows, which of course, until lockdown, were always live. At the start of each year I have worked with your producers, giving them twelve months of dates. This year in January I put your show dates in the diary, and I thought I was being overly optimistic putting them in till the end of June. Now that date has passed. How long should I enter them for? You said yesterday you're getting worse, but I think we both know that the shows are your lifeline. They give you a purpose, a reason to get up. When you stop them, you will probably soon stop yourself. I have put them in till the end of July. Four more weeks. I think I am being very cautious.

This was an issue most of all in January and February when you sounded worse than you do now. I'd ask if you wanted a break for a week; you said you'd never have the strength to return. Some shows took two days to record you were so puffed and exhausted. Since you 'came out' about your illness you seem to have got a new lease of life, ironically. You seem to feel freer and laugh on-air, calling yourself Puffing Billy – turning adversity into advantage.

Now, as I look back at the earlier months of this year, it makes me reflect on something you kept saying back then. You were fretting about a couple outside Wogan House on NYE. I wanted to do a video of you to put up on the socials before the show, so we went down to the entrance. The couple were waiting to see Michael Ball when he came out, so I let them know they were at the wrong studio, as he was coming from Maida Vale. I continued talking to you, suggesting where you should stand. 'Oh, are you famous?' they asked. I shared a laugh with you. Are you, Johnnie?! A penny dropped very slowly. The man asked if you were *that* Johnnie Walker? It seems you were. And while you weren't the prize they were after, they did remember you from your Radio 1 days (ha ha!) and wanted a photo with you as a consolation. You politely agreed and they snuck in close to you, grinning broadly. At least they had something to show the kids, even though it was clearly an enormous step down from Michael. We don't always get what we want.

Producer Paul has always protected you when you come to the studio. That day he wouldn't let the BA (broadcast assistant) come into the show, as she had a cold. You were exposed to just him and studio manager Jamie – both fighting fit. So the question that has stayed with you since is: did one of the mystery couple have Covid or a virus, and was that the blow that struck you down at New Year? Because without doubt you are stronger, healthier and less coldy now than you were back in January and February – the months when I thought you really would go any day.

Paul is in constant touch with me, telling me that it has to come from us, the decision to stop. And here we are in July. I do check with you most weeks if you're OK still doing the show, and yes, you are. Over the past two weeks your shows have been particularly good, and that gives you confidence. Indeed, since coming clean about your illness you are enjoying them more, which in turn feeds you. You always were contrary – 'I'm dying. Oh no I'm not!'

Our friend Dave Holmes arrives from the Isle of Wight. 'Just popping in to see how you are.' He asks the two nurses who are here doing a routine visit, 'Has he told you who I am?' He has not. 'I'm his undertaker!' They think it's a joke, but actually it's true. Dave told you years ago he'd do it for you. Once the nurses have left, you hit him with questions. What car will I be driven away in? What will be over me? What will I be wearing as I leave the house? Will I go in the fridge? Can Tigs visit me? Can I have Bruce Springsteen's 'Born to Run' blasting from speakers in the hearse? Is it OK for me to go to the crematorium in Salisbury alone while the wake happens? Dave answers everything with his usual reassuring calmness.

GT, our accountant is coming to check that we have everything in order, and he wants to see you. You start proceedings. 'How will Tigs survive?' GT and I go back decades. I was one of his first clients when he opened his own accountancy firm and I opened my production company Wowhaus. We were brave newbies together.

GT looks at you and tells you not to worry. I am resourceful, a survivor. He turns to me and tells me I need to work again – music to my ears. He tells us both I need to sell the Primrose Hill flat. It's not necessarily my ideal decision – I crave more culture – but as GT says, I don't need to own an expensive asset to spend under fifty nights a year in the Big Smoke. I need to simplify my life. He is, and always will be, my voice of reason.

He looks over your will. He asks about your assets. We all laugh – there are none. The property is in my name, and your pension is tiny. You never were good with money. Fantastic at spending it; less good at holding on to it. I have always squirrelled money away to pay for our holidays. I am squirrelling now to keep us going should you need to stop working. In a way I've secretly admired your carefree attitude, though I couldn't remotely be like that myself. Life – it's all a big board game, isn't it? And we all have different ways of playing it.

This time has become a marathon and I am a sprinter. This endurance race is depleting all my reserves and shows no sign of stopping. That is the dilemma of this period. I love you, I want to care for you, but it is exhausting me. Not so much the physical side; I can bathe and dress you, empty pee bottles and commodes, and grab oxygen tubes on top of cooking, cleaning, gardening, doing the bins, shopping, making beds, running the home and our lives as well as anyone. I have realised with the guidance of my longstanding homeopath, Carole, that my tiredness is mainly emotional and spiritual. In essence, I feel trapped. I'm not free to go away, to plan my life, to find my power. My focus is almost exclusively on your needs. I want to be in control and, thus, the greatest gift I could be given would be for someone to tell me when this will end, because then I could adjust my mental thinking accordingly. This is a marathon now, but is it actually a double marathon? Will you outlive me? Not that old chestnut again.

We discuss why you are holding on. I quote a friend who said quite matter-of-factly, 'Of course he's holding on, because you look after him so well. He's fed, washed, cared for, forgiven and thousands of people are sending him love. Who wouldn't hold on for that?'

Who isn't fed by love? Your listeners idolise you. Some idolise *us*, saying what an amazing inspirational couple we are. Us? WHY? I'd say we're as flawed as the next couple.

Apart from giving me a remedy and telling me to keep off coffee for three days, Carole's advice is that I have to live in the NOW. She fears that all the time I'm planning my future – be it where I'll live, my film or how to keep going financially – I am affecting your soul. Maybe you aren't letting go because I'm not at peace. She tells me to let go, to stop fretting about your end date and just embrace each day. She knows I'll be heartbroken, but she recognises more the fatigue. I must change my mantra, stop saying how tired I am, and just appreciate the good moments we have left.

I am more relaxed by the time I'm home from seeing her. I try to lasso you with your oxygen pipe. I hide the cuckoo bell you use to summon me in my top so my stomach appears to call like a bird when you press the button. I avoid any negatives. I make a chicken pie. You see I'm trying my new 'live in the moment' mantra, and in return hold my hand tightly at bedtime. You look small. It's such a struggle, you remind me.

Despite my determination to change for the better, my resolve to stay positive lasts thirty-two hours before I break down. My throat is swollen, I'm exhausted after a sleepless, fretful night and I haven't stopped all day. I feel like a servant, and you are, as ever, within your bubble. I force a flare-up and remind you that it cannot go on like this. I need help. But, of course, neither of us knows just what or how or who that help should be. I cry that I don't want our last months together to be miserable because I am so spent. I don't want to be angry that I have to do so much while you seem to be having a great time in bed or on your blue chair. I want us to have a good end. Not just you. Us. I deserve that after the sacrifices I've made. For the first time in my life I wish I had a child of my own who would come and help me, take the pressure off, give me time out or make me a cup of tea. I am hungry to be looked after for a while. Your son Sam would be here in a heartbeat if he didn't live in Australia. My mother has sent me a sheet of handwritten prayers, but right now I need something more tangible.

One of the things that really gets to me is that you never leave the house – you've hardly left it on your own since lockdown. And every married woman I know likes time alone in her home. I become a different person when you're not here. I listen to music you hate. I dance around. I make everything look beautiful. Just so. There's no farting, or empty coffee cups to pick up. But I cannot be alone in my home until you go. I have to leave the building to relax – which is really not what I always want at all. Of course, when you do next leave me alone in the house it will be in perpetuity, which isn't what I want either. I've always enjoyed you coming home.

You have had a lot of medical challenges during our marriage. Cancer, peritonitis, having much of your gut removed, stoma reversal op, tinnitus clinic (in Estonia!), stents, hospitalisation for various complaints, including pneumonia at least twice, heart attack, triple heart bypass, new knee, eyes lasered, eye lenses replaced and a lot of dental stuff. It has been fairly ongoing, and within these events I have faced the prospect of you dying more than once. Indeed, when you had an emergency operation for the peritonitis you stopped living three times on the operating table, but you came back, showing me early on in our time together that you are Captain Scarlet – indestructible. You've often talked about the film *They Shoot Horses, Don't They?* Well, I think you and I are one of the last couples on that dance floor, clinging to each other, still moving – just.

THE GOOD, THE BAD AND THE FAMOUS

Fame is an odd thing if you've never been exposed to it. The fabulous thing about you is that you never considered yourself famous. You were a radio jock, not a television presenter. You had the perfect situation. You had the influence of fame without the day-to-day recognition.

By and large fame was beneficial to us, though not at the start when I felt hopelessly out of my depth. I soon realised that you are all in a fame club (no matter what you are famous for) and some in that club are wary of outsiders. Do you remember the time you introduced me to Sharon Osbourne at the Elton John tribute? I told her she looked lovely, and she looked me up and down like a piece of shit, her face saying, 'How dare you address me directly.' Then I spoke to Billy Connolly; his silent look said the same. When you introduced me to Jeremy Clarkson at the Goodwood Festival of Speed it was a similar reaction. Just because you're famous does not mean you have manners – though of course you always did. On the few occasions you were noticed when you didn't want to be, for example because you were just about to eat fish and chips in a pub, you'd just turn to the person – chips on fork – and say, 'I'm off-duty, mate.' They always respected that.

There's no doubt that fame opens doors: to theatre and film openings, to festivals and of course to concerts. I mean, the list of musicians I've met with you is pretty starry: Elton John, Jackson Browne, Roger Daltrey, Robert Plant, Bonnie Raitt, the Dixie Chicks (all three), Mick Fleetwood, Neil Finn, James Taylor, Charles Esten, old timers Frankie Valli and Andy Williams, Christine McVie, Lulu and so many more. But nothing and no one will ever beat the time you introduced me to my hero, David Bowie. I've been crazy about him since the age of twelve, so I could never have imagined that event occurring. It was a Radio 2 gig (God bless that station) at Maida Vale. We swept up on your yellow Fatboy Harley-Davidson (which, for me, was quite a wild entrance). After the gig for around a hundred people, you talked your way backstage, where we were absolutely not invited – that privilege was for the Alan Yentobs of this world, but you got us back there – and as Bowie stepped out of the meet-and-greet with the great and the good of the BBC, you stepped forward, introduced yourself and quickly passed his attention to me. I said, overawed, 'I don't know what to say.' And Bowie, mirroring me, said, 'Neither do I' as if he too was overawed to meet me. I spoke about his set list. I loved that he'd played 'The Bewlay Brothers'. He seemed pleased. We probably only spoke for two minutes, but in those two minutes there was no one else that mattered in his life – or mine. He was fully present with me. Nothing else existed and it made me feel extraordinary. Had he always had that talent or did he learn it? It made him feel as powerful as I imagine Jesus Christ was. It's an awful thing to say to you, that it was almost the greatest moment of my life. The only moment to beat it was our first kiss. Those two events have in common that they were not mere earthly occurrences. Something other happened. Something spiritual and outside my body. They were both touched by God.

We have since talked often about Bowie and his power, not just as a musician, but as a man so visionary that I question whether he was man – or alien. To this day I know we have not seen the last of him. Whether as a hologram, or something not yet invented, I know he will come again. That suggests I'm saying he was Jesus Christ, and I don't think that. But he was beyond human.

One of my prouder starlit moments with you was when you introduced Bruce Springsteen on stage at St Luke's Church in the East End of London when he was doing that fabulous Seeger Sessions tour in 2006. It was being recorded for Radio 2 (again). The venue was small (again), and I sat with my former boss, James Studholme, in the side balcony. I was scared that you would falter in your duty; James reassured me that you would be fine. You did your bit, and I could hear in your voice the enormity of the event. Even though you've interviewed him several times, this was your musical hero, an artist you had lauded for years, and you were in front of an audience. Before you knew it, you'd delivered your intro and your hero was coming on stage with his guitar, saying, 'Thank you, Johnnie,' before he shouted out, 'One, two, three, four …!' and the band burst into song. Jeepers, what a moment. Talk about a proud wife.

Then there was backstage at the Round House when Elton did a Radio 2 gig. There was backstage, where all the bigwigs went, and then there was the real backstage – the inner sanctum of Elton's space. That's where we went – the only two invited in, as Elton wanted to see you. You, he and Ray Cooper (percussionist extraordinaire) sat on an L-shaped sofa. You told Elton he now had more hair than you these days, and Elton responded that he should do for the money it cost. The three of you reminisced and laughed. On the other side of the room was David Furnish and his friends. He totally ignored me. So there I was, standing in the middle of this room, feeling a total misfit. I didn't know where to put myself. Was I supposed to laugh at you three on the sofa? I smiled politely a lot until, happily, you'd had enough. In fairness, you were hugely apologetic that I'd stood there feeling like an idiot, though you didn't think I looked like one.

Your favourite story by far, and the one you told on your *Sounds of the 70s* show with huge amusement, was my faux pas at the Who concert at the Royal Albert Hall in aid of the Teenage Cancer Trust. Roger Daltrey had invited you/ us to be in his box with his wife and some other friends. As we sat there waiting for the gig to start I became aware of two men talking behind us. One was clearly a close friend of Mick Jagger as he mentioned him many times. The man with him had the most fabulous mane of hair. It's possibly a fault of mine, but I do pay people compliments (unless they are Sharon Osbourne), so I said to him how I loved his hair and that it gave him a look of power and strength. He really had something about him. He seemed pleased. After I turned back to you, I overheard him telling Mick Jagger's friend that he had never played at the Royal Albert Hall. It seemed rather cocky to me, but of course I was intrigued. I turned back again, 'Are you in a band?' He was. I asked which one, hoping like mad I would have heard of it. 'U2,' was his response. 'Fuck!' was mine. It was Adam Clayton, the bass player. Now, in fairness, he said that no one recognised him with the hair, which he had grown over lockdown, and he was loving being able to travel on the Tube. You didn't recognise him either, and it certainly gave the folks at Radio 2 a titter. It reminded me of the American tourist walking through the Scottish Highlands who bumped into our late, great monarch and asked her if she had ever met the queen. She said she had not but that her companion had. He asked her to take a photo of him with her companion. The queen never let on a word about who she was.

If there's one story I will tell as an old lady, it will be about the musician we met who hadn't yet found fame — although he was still trying in his late sixties. One day you turned to me and said, 'I want to go to a pub in Glastonbury on Thursday evening to see a band.' A pub? It clearly wasn't anyone big. You had read in the music press – *MOJO*, I think – someone raving about the greatest undiscovered rocker out there: Willie Nile. Willie was known by all the musicians – The Who, Bruce, Bono, etc. – but while they had all made the BIG time, Willie was playing pubs and working men's clubs. Having read the article about him, you looked up his UK tour dates to find out he was playing near us in two days' time.

We packed up Martha the Motorhome, deciding to go on to Putsborough Sands the next day, and off we set in time to have supper at the pub. As we sat in the back bar you nudged me – 'There's the band.' It wasn't that astute of you. I mean, they were five guys dressed top to toe in black with New York accents. They were having their pre-gig meal. Once they had finished eating you walked over. 'I'm sorry to bother you, I just wanted to say hello. My name's Johnnie Walker.' The older guy with the jet-black quiff of hair looked at you, saying, 'You're shitting me.' You said you were not shitting him. 'You can't be …' Willie continued. After several attempts, you assured him that you were indeed called Johnnie Walker and that you were a radio DJ on BBC Radio 2. You said it with assurance. Willie looked to his UK tour manager, Mickie, then back at you. He was utterly stunned. That VERY morning when he'd got up he'd said to Mickie, 'There's one person in this country I need to get my music to. Johnnie Walker.' Mickie had responded that this was not an easy ask. At all. And yet ten hours later, there you stood, waiting to hear Willie play.

Without doubt it was the most magical of meetings, and from then on we became not just firm friends; you two were soul brothers. On future UK tours the whole band would come and stay with us for a night. I remember the night I had to do dinner for them – the head count was about twelve including Janice, their driver, and our friend Big Pete. I asked if there were any intolerances. Just a few – dairy, gluten, seafood, red meat, mushrooms, garlic, nuts, rice and spices. Ay ay ay! Willie apologised. A highly individualised antipasto plate per person was followed by a simple lemon chicken, pomme dauphinoise made with stock instead of cream, and a gluten-free cake with berries. And still Willie's Italian partner, Cristina, had to raid the fridge to satisfy her needs, bringing a pack of Prosciutto ham and a whole avocado to the table. Thank goodness the red wine flowed.

Willie has a spirit the like of which I've never known. He writes, he performs, he tours. His life is music. He's never made the big time, but he assures me he doesn't want that. Bruce Springsteen plays with him and the band at least once a year for a charity gig at Asbury Park, New Jersey. The Who had him as their support act at a gig last year. He just lives the dream without the trappings. He has a band of ardent fans who follow him round the world, and I would include ourselves in that. Be it the 100 Club in London or a gig in Milan, we've been there to see him. Once we drove down to Montepulciano in Tuscany to see him play in a particularly smart vineyard. What a trip! We christened our new white Fiat Spider Bianca to get there, me quaking in the passenger seat on the terrifyingly narrow motorways as I was way too close to the crash barrier for my liking. Cristina, a cool Italian rock photographer, shrugged. 'Sure, we all drive like crazy. It's in our DNA.' She wasn't wrong.

When you were due to take a sabbatical month from Radio 2 I had one of my best ideas to date: Willie should do your *Rock Show*. I threw the idea to him. It was such an outside chance, but taking the bull by the horns, Willie recorded an hour-long demo show. With my hand on my heart, I can say it was the best hour of radio never broadcast. It was funny, with stories from 'the Village' where Willie lives in New York. I loved the one about him bumping into Patti Smith at the launderette some years past. He just said, off-hand, 'All her clothes were black. What other colour is there?' It was brilliant, personal, full of great music and stories about musicians, because he knew them all. It didn't cut the mustard for Radio 2 controller Helen Thomas, but if I had a radio station, Willie Nile would most certainly be my *Rock Show* host.

You and Willie always recognised the spirit and strength in each other, united, of course, by music. And while I don't imagine he will ever get fame in the traditional rockstar sense, to me he walks with the heart of someone who could handle it. And not many can.

OUR TOP TEN GIGS TOGETHER

James Taylor at the Hammersmith Odeon

*My first backstage experience and the night a punter shouted over to
ask if I was Sally Traffic, and I responded that I bloody wasn't!*

David Bowie at Radio 2

The afternoon I met my hero. A highlight of my life.

Bruce Springsteen at St Luke's Church in East London

*My most nervous moment ever as you introduced
The Boss on stage.*

Neil Young and Bruce Springsteen from the side of
the Pyramid Stage at Glastonbury

*Despite being thrown off several times by the US roadcrew,
I still got there. An unparalleled privilege.*

Elton John at the Round House

*We were invited backstage – and then into the inner sanctum,
where I met Elton.*

Simon & Garfunkel at Hyde Park

*Just wow. We'd argued beforehand and didn't talk throughout.
But still. Just wow.*

REM at St James's Church, Piccadilly

*Just extraordinary to see them at the top of their game
in a small church.*

Eagles at Wembley

*Shared with our friends Anna and Steve from Tresco. A bold dresser,
I told Anna not to let me down. She wore a loud yellow suit.*

The Peter Green Tribute Concert at the Palladium

*The most star-studded line-up of guitarists ever at this hottest
of gigs just before lockdown.*

Bruce Springsteen in Dublin

*We thought it was his goodbye tour, but as it happens it was your
goodbye concert, not his. Never to be forgotten.*

NOW

THE BEGINNING
OF THE END

Last night a photo popped up on my phone of us having dinner at the Gurnard's Head in Cornwall. It was 21 December 2022. Our twentieth wedding anniversary. I looked fit and slim in my black cord boiler suit. You looked suitably tasty in jeans and my favourite navy-blue linen shirt. We had the table by the fire and enjoyed a good meal and a glass too many of wine. We were demob happy. In all your decades of work you'd never had a sabbatical, so I'd asked Radio 2 if you could take a month unpaid leave in January. They agreed readily. This was the first night of our time out. The night before going to our beloved Tresco for Christmas.

You've always preferred getting there by helicopter rather than plane – altogether more rock star. Six of us got into the chopper at Penzance Heliport. You were already on nightly oxygen so your freedom pass to go anywhere was your portable oxygen concentrator. You were asked to carry it on board because of the battery. We were so excited as we saw the first of the islands that make up the Isles of Scilly. I was quite anxious about it flying on time as I had an important Zoom meeting at 5 p.m. I told you that whatever happened I needed to be on that call, as I was meeting an important actress to talk about the lead role in my film.

We landed smoothly and on time. What happened next I remember in slow-motion. I got off the chopper first. I wanted to wait for you and hold your arm as you got off, but I was called forward because of the rotating blades. I just remember turning round to check that you were OK. As you stepped down I could see something wasn't too stable. You were clutching your oxygen machine hanging on your shoulder. It cost a lot (thousands!) and you couldn't survive without it. The step was small, and the poor guy who should have been helping you was getting a walking stick out of the hold for another customer who looked more unstable than you. It was a bad decision that the poor man has to live with.

'Oh, Johnnie,' I whimpered as I watched you fall to the ground below like a tree being felled. You were stiff and upright as you clung to the machine, trying to protect that rather than your head, which landed first and hard against the plastic honeycombed-shaped flooring below. You lay still. I'm not the only one who thought you were dead. The ground staff rushed towards you. A wheelchair appeared. Blood gushed from your forehead in a honeycomb shape. 'Oh, Johnnie,' I kept repeating. I still had to wait where I was because of the blades. To this day I question myself about this. I am so law abiding and well behaved – you might have been about to pass away, but I didn't move to be by your side, as I was told not to. Pussy.

We may have landed on an island with only 150 residents, but the rescue procedure could not be faulted. Within minutes a first responder was looking at your wound. The cut went down to the bone. He apologised but you would have to go to the main island of St Mary's where there is a cottage hospital. A Noddy-car ambulance drove us to the quay. As we waited for the boat our dear friend Anna appeared. 'Johnnie, that's a corker!' She clutched my hand. I was in deep shock; she saw that and said I had to stick with you, take our luggage and very possibly accept that we'd be in Truro hospital later. Our Christmas break had lasted all of ten minutes. Never did I think it would involve both a boat and land ambulance.

You know, Johnnie, you have brought a lot of drama to my life. A lot. And not always good drama. But you have also shown me how luck has been sprinkled across your life. You were very lucky that you were still alive. You were even more lucky that the nurse on duty had recently relocated to the island of St Mary's and was a trauma specialist. She had the ability to sew up very nasty wounds like yours. When we were told that the final boat back to Tresco was at 4.45 p.m. she sped up her sewing.

There were no taxis to be had. It was 22 December and they'd all broken up for Christmas. So the hospital staff bundled us and all our luggage back into the ambulance and rushed us down to St Mary's quay. We staggered down the steps to the last boat, you looking like a survivor from the First World War.

As the boat crashed across the waves I clung to my laptop and tried calling my casting director. Could she delay the actress meeting? No. The actress had family Christmas commitments. So producer Jayne-Ann had to start the meeting without me.

What a sight we were as we arrived at the New Inn pub where we were staying: you bandaged around your head and me gasping to get into our room to join the meeting. I was fifteen minutes late, and switched from desperate wife to film writer and director. The actress was charming and intelligent, with an innate strength. I shall never forget the day I met her.

The word on Tresco spread like wildfire – Johnnie Walker had thrown himself out of the helicopter head-first. Some asked, 'Why didn't he wait for it to land?' – I love the humour of those islanders. In truth, it meant that you lay in bed for much of the five-day break. I had huge stomping walks alone, and Christmas lunch for me was spent with thirty strangers – the other residents of the pub – while you slept in bed.

Without doubt, that accident was the start of your decline. As part of your sabbatical, we were next heading for three weeks in Grenada. As we arrived at reception you were coughing constantly and in a bad way. I asked if there was a nurses' station at the hotel. Mercifully there was and yet again we were put in a buggy to a medical facility the minute we arrived. Your pulse was 28bpm. I asked the nurse to use another machine as it was clearly faulty. She kindly obliged, but that too read 28bpm. I muttered that I didn't have the nerves left to go away with you again. An hour of heavy-duty oxygen and your pulse increased. We were taken to our room and instead of going out for dinner as I had dreamt about, I ate a room-service meal while you slept.

You were notable at the two resorts where we stayed in Grenada – you were the only person on the beach staggering around with a walking stick. It had become your much-needed prop since the fall. You couldn't get in the sea or walk very far. Of course, you were still the naughtiest resident at the hotel. As you were the almost-final guest in the pool bar late one evening, the smiling night staff had to take you in a buggy back to our room and help you to the door. While many, like me, would be embarrassed by this, you thought it was brilliant when I reminded you about it in the morning. I can see that look of pride in your eye. 'I may be seventy-seven but rock 'n' roll is alive and well, and I'm still one of its ambassadors. Despite the stick!' You are and will be a monkey till the day you die. It's one of the things everyone loves about you. Including me – most of the time.

That photo of us at the Gurnard's Head will always be precious to me. Though neither of us knew it, it was your last night of being a strutting, virile man. After that fall you started to become an old and frail one. It's been downhill ever since, and I so miss the man I last saw on the night of our twentieth wedding anniversary, and the life of fun we shared together.

An afterthought on dates. I have realised that everything dramatic you've done has been on significant dates, as if the stars were double aligned. You first fell ill on our honeymoon. You fell out of a helicopter the day after our big wedding anniversary, and this year you neatly deteriorated on 1 January. Subconsciously, you always choose significant dates. So that has got me wondering, will you decide to let go on a date that will give added dramatic impact? I rather think you might. So I've been racking my brains for the next days of import. If I were a bookie I would be giving short odds on your demise on the following dates:

14 August – the fifty-seventh anniversary of the Marine, Broadcasting (Offences) Act 1967, when you continued to broadcast on Radio Caroline, making you a criminal and a radio legend in one move.

20 August – five years to the day when your respiratory consultant, Rohan Mehta, said you had two to five years left.

7 September – to make sure you are the headline news at the Radio 2 in the Park weekend in Preston.

21 December – our twenty-second wedding anniversary.

25 December – just so I will always hate Christmas.

26 December – just so I will always hate my birthday even more than I already do.

1 January 2025 – just to make it a neat year since your final decline.

26 January 2025 – the final *Sounds of the 70s* show in your contract.

30 March 2025 – your eightieth birthday.

For verification, these dates are being predicted on 11 July 2024!

THEN

STARDUST

You so often apologised to me for being so ill/such a lot of work to keep afloat/so dominating in my life. Mainly when I got down about it. It wasn't your fault you were ill. It's just the way the dice rolled. Yes, you have dominated my life, but that's because that soul of mine that intertwined with yours when we first kissed accepted that I was going to play second fiddle to you and your career. I didn't consciously recognise it at the time, otherwise I would have run! But I am certain that's what happened. That said, I have often bitched about being lost and out of my power, which is why it's so important that, as you get weaker and the final curtain gets closer, we look back at the sprinklings of stardust that have peppered our marriage, at the many things that only happened because you are you. Let's pretend we're sitting across our dining-room table from each other. You have laid the table, lit the candles and opened a bottle of Chablis, while I have cooked us a healthy supper of trout fillet, cavolo nero (or 'hedge' as you call anything green) and sweet potato wedges – a fairly usual meal for us. As the first glass slips down, cool and delicious, our day floats away and our minds turn to some of our highlights together.

I'll start with the first Radio 2 Presenters' Christmas Dinner at the Reform Club in 2001. What a fabulous grand Pall Mall setting – back in the days before the budgets were slashed. Jim Moir was the controller. He was old school, with a fantastic touch for what and who worked well on the station. 'Evolution, not revolution' was always his mantra. At that dinner, so new into our relationship, you introduced me to Terry Wogan, who was charm itself. 'You're far too good for him,' he joshed with me as we walked up the grand staircase together. Then he added, 'The trouble with Johnnie is that he doesn't know how good *he* is.' How right. I sat next to Jeremy Vine at dinner. He was about to start on the station in the old Jimmy Young slot. I spoke to him, bemused that he would leave *Newsnight* – then the bastion of intelligent BBC journalism – to go to Radio 2. Why was he dumbing down? His answer was that he wanted his name on a show, and how right he proved to be.

I would never have gone to Glastonbury without you. It wasn't, as with many, a rite of passage I needed to go through before middle age. I just thought, *Why not?* The first time was magical as we stayed in a tipi in the Healing Fields. That area sits above the site and was a spiritual haven from the scrum below. We were with your old biking mate Snapper – a wild West Countryman if ever there was one. I woke the first morning to him squatting down next to me. 'Morning, Duchess. I've bought you a cuppa.' I opened my eyes to see that he was stark bollock naked. His pendulous manhood remains my dominant memory of that weekend. I couldn't face the tea. We returned a couple more times with Martha in the three years we had her. How good it was being AAA – access all areas. Being short, I struggle with big crowds and honestly refer to the festival as a war zone, but if you get to stand at the side of the Pyramid Stage watching the bands, that is a major dollop of privilege. I can go one further. You used to DJ on that stage between sets. You shared it with a local DJ, Chris Bull, who still does it to this day. When we went in 2009, we went to see Chris. For some reason you and he both asked me to put on a song, so I did: Oasis, 'Wonderwall'. What happened was beyond my belief. The thousands of people sitting on the grass in front of the stage got up and sang. I stared in amazement. So did you and Chris. 'How do we follow that?' you asked. It was the first time in my life, possibly the only, when I could see the power of music. I felt like a megalomaniac for the rest of the afternoon.

The Boat That Rocked film premiere in Leicester Square was pretty memorable too. Because you were the only pirate DJ there we were papped endlessly as we went down the red carpet. That was a new experience. I kept thinking, *Breathe in, weight on the back leg, smile*. While the film was a shocking representation of what it was actually like on Radio Caroline, it did bring that important piece of social history to the awareness of people around the world. At the end of the film, Philip Seymour Hoffman says, 'I realised we've just lived the best days of our lives.' You told director Richard Curtis you wished you'd thought of saying that when Radio Caroline actually did end. He graciously said he'd had forty-five years to come up with the line. The after-party was amazing. It's the only time I've stood just behind Paul McCartney, and I unashamedly shook Bill Nighy's hand just by the chocolate fountain.

Goodwood has over the years given us heaps of enjoyment at the Festival of Speed, the Revival, the Members' Meeting, Goodwood Racing and, one year, the Vintage Festival. Charles, then Lord March and now the Duke of Richmond, has to be one of the hardest-working, most stylish and dignified people in the world. And Janet, his wife, is a pure, down-to-earth delight – and a real duchess! (One of only twenty-four, excluding the royals.) As for their guest list, it has to be the best in Britain, if not the world. You never knew who you would be sat next to at dinner: racing drivers, actors, musicians or leading businessmen. The balls they throw are out of this world. One year the theme was Venice and they actually built a miniature Rialto Bridge to enter the enormous ballroom (located in a marquee). On a couple of occasions we were put up in Goodwood House itself, where for you the major attraction was not the incredible art collection, but the butler, Monty, and his impressive butler's table of drinks. How you would love to sink into one of the divine red velvet sofas in the drawing room at the end of an evening with a tipple. The first time we stayed was for the one-off Vintage Festival, at which you were broadcasting your *Sounds of the 70s* show live. The house got a bit overrun with guests, partly because some did not want to leave. I remember the actor Matt Smith being there with an entourage and them all demolishing the breakfast buffet. But the really memorable time was when we were put in the Queen's Room. Goodness. This was where Her Majesty would stay. The next day I said to Charles how honoured I felt that we had been put in the best room. 'I don't want to disappoint you, Tiggy, but there is a King's Room too, which is even better.' We were both amused.

Because it was known that you loved Formula 1, that led to a few great invites. For you, the best was Monaco and being shown round the pits before the race – that, and an amazing dinner on board an incredibly smart boat the night before. Privileges you cannot buy. I preferred our last time at Silverstone when we did the famous grid walk. Oh, the noise and power! I bumped into the *Strictly Come Dancing* professionals Janette Manrara and her sparkly husband Aljaž Škorjanec. He was as excited as me to be there. 'Just look where dancing has got you,' I observed. 'You're right,' he responded, as if I was some sort of sage.

There have been some incredible dinners. Your friend Mitch Tonks invited us to a special one at his restaurant the Seahorse in Dartmouth (our favourite eatery in the UK). The extraordinary and legendary butcher-cum-chef from Tuscany called Dario Cecchini was cooking with his team. What a night. We were sat with Robin and Judy Hutson who owned the Pig hotels (our favourite accommodations in the UK), and much hilarity was enjoyed by all. There is no doubt that the people who party best are chefs and hoteliers. There is a camaraderie between them, an understanding of what a tough business it is, and how much fun there is to be had when they take time out. The next morning Mitch took us in his boat from the Dart Marina Hotel to his Rockfish restaurant in Brixham. Eight of us had a memorable breakfast of brandy, white wine and John Dory.

As a result of that night Robin and Judy invited us to a couple of their Smoked and Uncut music festivals at their Pig hotels, the best moment being when you and actor Hugh Bonneville came to dinner wearing the same shirt.

As John and Steph Illsley were also there that night, a couple of months later we all had lunch at their stunning house on the Solent. I was sitting next to Mark Knopfler, lead singer of Dire Straits, who I love. What heart and soul he has. As we left that day he said to me he would do anything for you. That really touched my heart. My mother, on the other hand, has never been impressed by any of your showbiz trappings – except the Queen's Room at Goodwood – and meeting 'Lord Grantham', who I swear she has a bit of a crush on. I told Hugh Bonneville that he has a unique ability to make a ninety-two-year-old, highly respectable, deeply Christian woman somewhat fluttery. He looked at me with a totally straight face and said, 'It's why I went into showbiz.'

The Peter Green Tribute Show at the London Palladium on 25 February 2020 has to go down as one of the most body-tingling, star-studded rock gigs we ever went to. Tickets were like gold dust, and it was only thanks to having Mick Fleetwood on your show a couple of days previously that we managed to secure tickets. What a privilege. The line-up of artists included Billy Gibbons ('Is that beard for real?' I whispered in your ear), David Gilmour, Christine McVie, Jonny Lang, Kirk Hammett, Andy Fairweather Low, John Mayall, Zak Starkey, Steven Tyler, Bill Wyman, Mick Fleetwood, of course, who had pulled it together, and last but not least, Neil Finn, who came to find us afterwards – the last time you saw him. I have to admit that it was the only time in my life that I transcended out of my seat as Kirk Hammett from Metallica played with Billy Gibbons and Steve Tyler on his guitar, which had once belonged to Peter Green. It was simply sublime. Pulling all those artists together on the same night took huge amounts of planning and preparation. And as luck would have it, it happened just a few weeks before the world locked down for Covid.

All the special events that happened after the lockdowns had so much more weight to them, as we all felt so very grateful to be doing anything outside the house. Our final bit of glamour was the night you were asked to DJ at the Palace of Versailles near Paris in July 2023. To be honest, I was truly nervous to accept the gig for you. At this stage you could no longer get health insurance, and I was terrified that the pressure of performing in public would be too much for you. However, it was for Sir Jim Ratcliffe, who was throwing a party for his staff, and I knew you respected his business chutzpah. Plus, his brother, Bob, had been one of your motorbike gang in the past. Clearly the budget was not an issue. I was so chuffed that you were asked to do a one-hour set that I just said yes without even negotiating or telling them your health was dodgy. I wanted us both to experience the thrill of going to Versailles for what I knew would be your final public appearance. What a place to bow out! I would have paid *them*.

Beforehand we had heated rows about what should be on the set list, me feeling that, at sixteen years younger, I was a bit more in touch with what people would want to dance to. You insisted that 'Hi Ho Silver Lining' was always a hit on the dance floor. I told you that if you played that, the night would be a disaster. I hadn't heard it since my primary school days, and even then I thought it was pretty dubious. We brought one of your producers, Johnny Kalifornia, with us for technical back-up, insurance in case you should feel ill and for another opinion on songs. It was late by the time you did your set. Michael McIntyre had amused the guests between courses, a musical firework display reflecting in the formal Versailles ponds had given us all a thrill, Jools Holland and his band had played, and then finally it was your turn. As ever, I had that manager/wife set of nerves about whether people would like your choices. I slipped into the party to watch you. At the bar I met the most amazing woman called Fran Millar, who is the CEO of Belstaff. She couldn't believe I was your wife – I imagine because I was younger than you. I know she'd had a good evening, but still I'm not sure if I've ever felt as flattered as I did when this good-looking, fit, beautifully dressed and incredibly successful woman looked down at me and said, 'Tiggy, you are the woman I want to be one day.' Was it simply that I was sober? As she and I spoke, I heard the dreaded opening chords of 'Hi Ho Silver Lining'. I spun round and looked up at you. And you, my Johnnie, looked defiantly back with that 'I know what I'm fucking doing, baby' look that you saved for those times you were right and I was clearly wrong. For the dance floor not only filled with many dancers, but they started doing a form of the conga. Oh, how that thrilled you. I just had to laugh and acknowledge your DJing superiority.

I don't think stardust is dependent on fame, privilege, power or indeed palaces. We've had stardust in so many ways. Bobbing on a boat off Tresco with Steve and Anna who live on the island. Or driving Bianca to Ringstead Bay on the Dorset coast for a swim (me, not you!). Staying in a beach hut with Darcey Dog at Mudeford Sandbank. Having a Campari and soda at Roxi Bar in Loggos as the sun sets. Or dancing together in our kitchen to John Prine's 'All the Way With You'. We have been blessed.

The bottle of Chablis is empty, and you suggest a glass of red and a bit of cheese, plus a couple of batons of Hotel Chocolat 70 per cent. We've always known how to have a great evening together. Good food, good wine, good memories, laughter. What extraordinary companions we have been to each other.

You add, 'If there's one email I wish I'd kept, it's the one from the man who named you Tiggy Stardust. Why didn't we ever think of that name for you?'

Because, my darling Duke, we're not the kind of people to call ourselves 'Stardust'. While it was delightful that he did, we're just a couple who enjoy the sparkle on those few occasions it's been sprinkled on us. We just possibly had more than our fair share.

TEN SONGS I'D LIKE TO PLAY FOR YOU

You always loved it when I had a song-playing session for you. You really enjoyed hearing my choices. These are selected for you, now you're on high.

Tom Baxter
THIS BOY

For you knew how to stand up after falling down.

Neil Diamond
MAN OF GOD

You were.

Glen Campbell
THESE DAYS
Such a beautiful rendition of this Jackson Browne song,
and captures the gentle decline of a music man.

Jackson Browne
THE LOAD OUT
A wonderful song about the end of a show as it's
all packed away ...

Pink Floyd
GREAT GIG IN THE SKY
I bet that's what you're having up there.

Emmylou Harris
GOODBYE
Because I never said those words at the end.
I called an ambulance instead.

Bruce Springsteen
WILD HORSES
You were chasing 'wild horses', especially as a young man.
We loved his film Western Stars with his profound,
soulful voiceovers.

Joan as Police Woman
ETERNAL FLAME
Fantastic song, and my flame for you is eternal.

Elton John and Brandi Carlile
DO YOU BELIEVE IN ANGELS?

This is the one song since you died that I know you would have loved. Their voices together are sublime. I really want you to hear it. I saw them perform it together at The Palladium thanks to your dear boss Helen.

Mark Knopfler
GOING HOME: THEME OF THE LOCAL HERO

Because it's one of the best ever tracks to end a film and it will fill you full of hope that one day we'll be together again. Just like in the movies …

NOW

YOU'VE GOT A FRIEND (OR TWO)

After some days of emotion (mine, not yours), just possibly the homeopathy is working its magic. That or having a day off has done it. I've been to London – for lunch with girl-friends, one of whom is over from Seattle. We eat at Spring in Somerset House, a delightfully light and airy restaurant with delicious food. I look around at the clientele and think, *This is more like it*. An urban fix, girlfriends, honest chat and Chablis. It is absolutely what I need. I return so brimming with life and excitement that you don't recognise me from yesterday. I bring good energy back to the house, while you have two messages you want to share. Daniel Cainer has written you a song using your mantra, 'No amount of worrying ever changed tomorrow.' And Peter Kay has left you an amazing voice note about our podcast and your shows. He tells you that *Sounds of the 70s* is your purpose and that you must go on doing it, and he asks how I am. He says it must be tough for me. Bless him for think-ing of me, and caring. I've never met him, but he's always been so kind to you.

The thing about having so many guests these days is that we're not getting that much time just for us to be together. This is our time. A profound, special, limited time. But others want a piece of that. Of course they do. They want to see you, tell you nice things, say goodbye. In these six months we have seen more people at our home than we have in our entire marriage. This week no fewer than nineteen people are visiting. It is the main thing that is robbing me of my strength. It's a lot of tea, coffee, wine, biscuits, cakes, soups and salads to prep. Plus I have to tidy the house every time, make sure you're up and dressed, and occasionally bathed like today. And when you don't feel like talking, I have to. Often you fall asleep in front of them. I lose hours and hours of my life making small talk when I should be doing stuff. The garden is suffering from neglect.

Of course, friends are so valuable. And to you, they are the only thing that significantly changes your world from one day to the next. They bring news and gossip, energy, ideas, memories, laughs. I feel they are important for you. It is wonderful that so many people care.

I have had a rule for a couple of months that if you want to come for supper, you cook it. We have our 'gang of six' – d'Arcy, Gary, Jane and Charles – and the only way we can meet up together is for everyone to come to ours. D'Arcy does a three-course meal that we all devour. There's much chatter and hilarity around the table, but you reverse in your wheelchair away from the table. You can't quite cope with it all. Later I find you outside having a fag with your cannula blowing oxygen up your nose. You don't care. I'm really shocked. It is the only time in twenty-two and a half years that you have blatantly smoked in front of me. It's a real 'fuck it' statement. You retire to bed, our guests leave and at midnight, when I finish tidying up, I fall asleep fully clothed on my bed. The open smoking feels like a deliberate slap in the face to me. I just keel over. I wake in the morning in a crumpled new Toast shirt with mascara down my face. That, I feel, should be our last supper event. I'm not saying that to protect you, but myself.

Next day your friend Mike comes to lunch. His jumper is on the sofa, but he is not. I ask where he is. You have sent this poor man from London, who has no satnav or Google Maps, to go and buy you a pack of cigarettes, as no one else will. Poor Mike is gone for over thirty minutes, totally lost in deepest rural Dorset. You're on another planet if you think I don't care anymore about you smoking. I tell you that's fine if you want to smoke, but I don't have the strength to care for someone I don't respect. I make an appointment at the local care home, which I am going to check out the week after next. This shocks you and elates me. I'm finally acting on what the medium Jean said – that you would be better off in a home. I suddenly realise that you can be a part of my life without me being trapped by the caring. I can sell this house. Go somewhere I love. Not be constantly knackered and frustrated. I see light at the end of the very long, dark tunnel I am in. You tell me you hate the idea, that you want to keep doing your show. That really is your trump card. I can hardly put you in a home with half your room taken up with a studio set-up. But the thought of being free … it gives me the hugest sense of hope. And a bit of a thrill to be honest. I have not become a total bitch. I am at the end of my tether. I know I am no fun to be with. I go through the motions of daily life, but I'm not engaging in it or enjoying myself. I am sure a break from me would be as healthy for you as it would for me.

I am getting more sluggish by the day. I told my fitness instructor this morning that in the past four weeks I've gained 5kg. FIVE KILOS! How? I exercise six days a week. I don't think my habits have changed. But then you just have to remember what goes with guests: cake, wine, gin, crisps … She says the perfect thing to me: that I cannot worry about my weight right now. I'll have plenty of time to get myself back together, and I know she will be only too happy to be part of that betterment of Tig. I am surrounded by some wonderful women who are all there, ready to catch me.

I am not alone in my depletion, though. You are wrung out too. At bedtime you tell me you've had enough. It is all such an enormous effort for you. When I help take off your jogging pants as you lie on your bed, you need a minute's break to regain your breath before I put on your pyjamas. Your oxygen goes down to 62; 90 is the lowest it should be. Every night, and indeed many times during the day, you test your oxygen level with your oximeter. It's the best phys- ical indicator of how much your body is struggling. At bedtime we always wait for you to recover to at least 80 before turning the oxygen concentrator down a few notches for the night. Most of the day it's on maximum, as the smallest physical effort now slaughters you. The question arises, why are you taking so many pills to keep you going? Steroids, statins, blood thinners … Plus I load you up with vitamins and minerals to keep you strong. Perhaps we should cut some back. We agree we will talk to Angel Caroline about all this and what you can safely drop.

A friend contacts me after a visit. They are worried about me, and honestly, I'm a little worried about me. I am not coping too well. I'm feeling a bit unhinged. Worrying more about me than you. And my dreams are insane.

I recognise the similar symptoms to when I went through chemo – not knowing when it would end, not being able to plan and drive things forward, not travelling, having no control, feeling trapped by the situation. I was offered counselling when I was prescribed my antidepressants in March. At the time I laughed. I don't need that! I just need to stop crying and regain some energy. But now I think I do need counselling. It's not a weakness. The weakness would be if I crumbled altogether. Then what use am I to either of us?

I am lucky. The GP surgery answers my online request for help quickly. Within a day I'm talking to a counsellor on the phone, and she offers me six weeks of free sessions starting next week. She realises I just need to be heard, to vent. I do.

It's great timing as ten minutes later I'm talking to Fi Glover for Times Radio. Just the knowledge that I'm getting some help gives me strength. She asks if you're still rock 'n' roll. I tell her that you've started smoking the odd cigarette. I make it funny, but even so, I get post-interview remorse wishing I'd not said it, as it was not only a betrayal of confidence, but also I made it sound like I find it funny, which I don't at all.

John and Jackie Inverdale are visiting when the interview goes out. We get all the inside chat from Wimbledon where for the first time John had gone as a punter, not a commentator – after a thirty-nine-year stint. You remind him of your favourite moment of him commentating there: the famous rainy day, pre the Centre Court roof, when Cliff Richard got hold of a mic and started singing 'Summer Holiday'. The despondent crowd loved it. Cliff, encouraged, went on to sing another. And another. John, you remind him, said sardonically, 'You're listening to Cliff Richard's fifty greatest hits. Only forty-seven more to go.' John is a good guest. Entertaining. Interesting. He used to dep for you on *Drivetime*, including the period between you being taken off the show and Chris Evans starting. There's always a buffer presenter to lessen the shock of the new person starting. In huge loyalty to you, when John signed off his final show on the Friday before Chris started, he ended with the words, 'This is the end of an era. From Monday, the world is orange.' He wasn't booked by Radio 2 again for a long time, but for you and your millions of fans, outraged at the change, it was a fantastic 'up yours' to the controller Lesley Douglas, who had fired you in order to get Chris into the station.

Not only do I enjoy the Inverdales' company, I'm relieved to be missing the Times Radio interview. I'm scared you'll be upset with me for being indiscreet about your smoking. I mean, it doesn't sound good, does it – dying of lung disease and smoking? Personally, I'd feel ashamed. When they leave I say I don't want to hear it back, so you listen on your own when I'm out of earshot. Later you tell me I'm really good. You think I covered a lot of bases, including politics, though that's a subject I try to avoid. I even got in a few statistics about carers. You don't mention the smoking reference. It was my first national radio interview alone about caring. Usually, I can just be your fall guy, letting you do the serious, professional, on-point bits, so your praise means a lot to me.

When I listen back I can hear Fi Glover trying to break in. Dear God – I go on and on. Like it's a therapy session. Carers UK get in touch and are very happy, but even more important is that a woman called Lucasta sends me a private message on Instagram. She thanks me for my honesty and tells me about caring for her dad, who was dying from cancer and living in her sitting room while she juggled her four kids. She ended up putting him in a care home for the time he had left and has felt guilty ever since. She said that listening to me gave her the first modicum of peace since that decision. This blows me away. Bless you, Lucasta. And

I am sure your dad blesses you for caring for him for so long.

Well, *Hello, Dolly!* You've arranged seats for me to see Imelda Staunton in this fabulous musical revival. I return to you as quickly as I can in the morning. When I get back you are laid out on your bed, in pyjamas, unhappy and exhausted. You may have sent me lovely texts while I was gone, but you have had the worst night on the loo and you didn't want me to know. What set you off? You haven't eaten the food I left for you. Or taken your pills. You are weak. You remain in bed, and I feel guilty for my twenty-four hours of stimulation and freedom. You tell me you fall apart when I am not there, and I fear deeply for my week off in France, which starts in ten days.

The next day you are still weak and exhausted. You have gone down a notch. It's the morning that the vicar Helen is coming to give us Communion, and joining her is Simon Everett, the vicar who married us. It's the second time we're having Communion at home, and while you're not a regular church-goer at all, it brings you comfort and allows Helen, who will do your funeral, to get to know you a bit more. You assure me you want to get up for it, but when I return from my exercise class you are fast asleep. I take an executive decision. I tidy your clothes away and arrange chairs around your bed. We will have Communion there. Your chest of drawers becomes an altar, as Helen gets out her doll-sized silver wine goblet and candle. As she starts reading the service I feel tears stinging my eyes because there's such comfort in the words, and something in me lets go like a child. You may be in bed, but your voice is strong as you say the prayers. I love it. No hymns, no sermon, just the words and Sacrament. There's surely a wider market than the infirm for speedy at-home Communions.

On a hot Sunday afternoon I smell smoke. This time you are not the cause. Our neighbour has lit a bonfire just the other side of the fence. I have to close every window and door to protect your lungs. Our main room gets to 26.5 degrees. You call to me, hot and claustrophobic. You need Oramorph. You are panicking. You beg me not to leave you, to hold you. Your oxygen level plummets. I put on your face mask so you can breathe through your nose. When you have calmed you tell me it was the closest to death you have come. Our home still stinks of smoke when I go to bed. If you die tonight, I'm getting our neighbour for manslaughter.

'You are the story that you tell.' These were the wisest, most healing words I was given by a former Buddhist monk when we once holidayed at Kamalaya on Koh Samui. At that time I had been telling a story of deep hurt about your ex. I stopped telling that story and the hurt disappeared. I notice your story has changed in the past week. We have been screening guests to ensure they are not carrying any infection. If you should catch a virus, chest infection or Covid then your story would come to an abrupt end. You would 'drop like a stone' is what Angel Caroline has always said. An awareness of that danger has been in the back of my mind all year. You may slowly and gracefully deteriorate, or you may suddenly go. Needless to say, you have always favoured the former route. However, the story you're telling now is that it is all too much effort. Putting on a shirt, getting into your wheelchair, cleaning your teeth … these have all been added to the challenge of going to the loo. The only places you are stress-free are your blue chair and bed. All the bits in between are so very tough on you and your lungs. You have almost had enough now, and thus you have started saying, partly in jest yet partly in all seriousness, if someone is sick, bring them in. You're getting ready to drop like a stone, and are starting to think this may be the best way to go.

Bruce Springsteen is playing Wembley on Thursday night. A friend texts that she's sure we could get you accessible tickets. I love her positivity that you could leave the house for this. Bruce was the last gig we went to, in April 2023 in Dublin, with our Irish friends Tommy and Mairead. Mairead is the wild one of their marriage, like you. When we were waiting at the airport I said to her, 'What would happen if you and Johnnie were a couple?' She quickfire replied, 'The first thing we'd do is rob a bank!' My God, how we laughed. It was 11.30 a.m. and you'd already ordered a round of espresso martinis. Dublin was a great place to see Bruce and the band. The RDS Arena is so much smaller than Wembley. It was a beautiful evening, the crowd was brilliant and Bruce was on form. He loves Ireland and that came through. When he ended the show alone on stage with a single spotlight on him and his acoustic guitar, and he sang that 'I'll see you in my dreams', it felt like a farewell. It certainly was yours (and later those lyrics would be spoken at your funeral by and at the suggestion of our friend Jane).

I'm terrified. I have a bad feeling in my chest. You have slept almost all day. Whenever you wake you seem a bit discombobulated. You leave nearly all the food and drink I bring you. You get up for about thirty minutes, but otherwise you're in bed sleeping. This is a first. You're just wiped out. I've been checking on you every half-hour since 5.30 p.m. It is the first evening that I have realised you really will die, that my evenings will always be this quiet. Johnnie, darling, I'm scared. I have to do the next bit without you.

What a night. I wake at 11.45 p.m. and go to check on you. I've left your bedroom door open so I can hear anything. The oxygen machine keeps going whether you're breathing or not, so that drones on all the time. I gingerly walk over to you lying on your side, facing the opposite wall. You're not moving. I can't see you breathing. I move closer and touch your skin. It's cool, clammy. You are breathing but so lightly that your body doesn't appear to move. I return to my room and google signs of near death. I conclude you have a few. I pray for you and fall back into a fitful sleep.

A nightmare wakes me. It's 3.45 a.m. I am certain this means you have passed. I lie there wondering whether I should just leave you as you are because there's no one I can call at this hour, or whether I should check on you. I decide ultimately that I have to go in to see you. And there you lie, like a perfect stone effigy on a tabletop tomb, your arms folded neatly across your chest, your face looking up to heaven. I admire you for your perfect end-of-it-all placement. My Duke. Lying there in peace. I lean in closer. And suddenly you lift one hand to rub your nose! You open your eyes. 'What are you doing in here?' You throw back your duvet and tell me to get in. Together, in your small four-foot divan bed, we settle down, trying to remember where we put our arms and bodies when we sleep together. It has been so long. We sleep for a few blissful hours. When we wake you ask rather critically why I didn't wake you up for supper last night. As if I had cooked. I just finished off scraps and felt sad.

Fear goes straight to your body. I return to my bed and sleep for hours – past the time when I should have left for my weekly Tuesday-morning yoga class. But it doesn't matter. My whole body feels as if it has just been in the boxing ring. I ache. I am weak. There's no way I could do chaturanga today. It will be a very small day, but I must cook some nutritional meals and get them down you.

I have used and abused my friends and my brother Martin and his wife, Kate, quite enough. They have all looked after you in times of my few absences. For the France week I decide that I should pay a carer for the majority of it. Butch (not his real name) used to be in hospitality but has taken up caring. We've known him for years and he is utterly charming. When I brief him in advance I jokingly say, 'No drugs, Butch!' A week later I am telling a friend that I've booked him, and she looks at me askance. 'You do know he had a huge cocaine habit.' We roar with laughter at both my 'No drugs' line to him, and me booking a former coke user to look after a former coke user. I go back home and tell you how funny this is.

'When you say goodbye on Sunday you must say it as if it is the last time you will see Johnnie. Anything could happen while you're away, so you must be prepared for that or you will suffer later on. If he's still here when you return, it will be a bonus.' These are the rather alarming but well-intentioned words from palliative nurse Angel Caroline before I go away.

And when I do look at you as I am about to leave for my respite week in France, your eyes are wide and healthy, sparkling at me. 'I think it will be as good for you to have a break from me as it is for me to go and have a rest,' I say. You don't respond to that, but you do say with confidence, 'I believe I will be here on your return.' I say I believe you will too. There are no tears. Just a hug. You wheel round to the front door to watch me depart. 'I love your arse.' I ask you to say no more. If those are the last words you ever say to me, I can live with it. It would be such a 'you' final comment, as you love that word. 'Arse.'

Driving to the station, I almost turn back. What am I doing? Our days together are numbered. Why am I deliberately spending some of them apart from you? But I remind myself, it is quality, not quantity, that always matters. I am shattered on every level, and I need to replenish so that our final time together can be better. I love you for understanding that, and seeing the profound need in me to rest.

You don't call me once while I'm gone. I always need to know you have woken, though, so you just text me 'Blues Song xx'. ('Well, I woke up this morning …') You share what you are being served for supper, none of which is a surprise as I either made or bought it all.

My time with my friends Camilla and Amanda in France is beyond precious. I have little to give. We swim, read, go to the village bar, visit markets, eat delicious food at the house. I am removed from the everyday stress. There's nothing I can do for you. Camilla kindly cooks most of the meals, although we all favour suppers of crevettes, salad and fresh baguette. After a week I feel a weight lift off me and a relaxation return to my face.

I return to you renewed. It wasn't just a life saver. It was an 'us' saver. My mindset shifts from you being my heavy burden of a charge who I have to do things for all the time, wondering when this will end, to a remembrance of the fact that I love you and you are my soulmate. I can see your deterioration in the time I was away. I sense that your time is chasing on. So do you. You are sleeping so very much more.

The greatest surprise of my break was your text saying you want a final disco at home. A kitchen wheelchair disco. You send the message when Butch is with you as he stays for dinner and a bottle of wine with you each night. You repay him with a song session, and with that, JohnnieFest is born. I double-check the next morning that it's really what you want. It is, so I will make it happen. Fifty mainly local friends are coming, plus your boss, Helen Thomas. I only quipped with her about it saying, 'Do come' – and she is. So is Mark Goodier, who of all your fellow jocks has always been the kindest and most supportive to us, including delivering us unbelievable food parcels from Ottolenghi, which has given our entertaining a touch of class that would otherwise have been missing.

I'm expecting JohnnieFest to be historic. It will certainly be your final blast on a dance floor. In a way it's your crescendo, but will it be your final act? It's your night. I want it to be everything you hope for, but I also know you want to push the boundaries. You've told me you're going to smoke openly. Fine. And drink a lot. Fine. But there's a further glint in your eye. We have our first spat in months.

'You can't!' I tell you.

'It's my night, you told me.'

'But, Johnnie, if you take drugs you might die. In front of everyone.'

'I won't.'

'You don't know.'

I know what you're doing. You're pushing your boundaries. Your rock 'n' roll heart wants to believe it can be truly naughty again. You want to make believe that you're young and carefree again.

It *is* your night, and I want you to be happy, but I also ask you to remember that we're throwing a party – with guests, so IF you should do something that your weak body cannot tolerate, I ask that you do so past ten o'clock so people will have had a couple of hours of dancing first. And don't, whatever you do, let me realise. And don't do anything to me, like you did at your seventieth-birthday dinner and knees-up when you slipped a tab of MDMA into my unsuspecting mouth. 'It's the Love Drug!' you cheered with drunken glee. I'm not sure about 'love' but I was certainly wired till the early hours and hated it. In fairness, you were utterly repentant later on.

I cannot deny, I am a bit anxious that you are serious about finding some form of non-NHS drugs and that these might finish you off. Equally, a tiny bit of me thinks that if you do, and it does finish you off – what a great way for Johnnie Walker, rebel to the end, to go. It would be so you (even though all the actual rock 'n' rollers these days seem to be as clean as a whistle). It's five days away and I do wonder what lies ahead. In the meantime, I'm ordering festoon lights and wine, and planning what nibbles to serve.

You wanted a kitchen disco and by God you're getting one. I ask you all week if you're up to it. You say you are, but my anxiety grows. I keep saying we can cancel but you don't want to. You want your night. You ask me to email our guests asking for requests. They come in thick and fast. Some great dance tracks, some that you wouldn't even get out of bed for. You compile the best on your iPad and mix them up with your own choices. I check that you have some Stevie Wonder and James Brown, but I don't get involved; the music is the one area I can delegate to you. That and turning on your disco light. I have enough to do with booze, food and lights.

For the few days before I am up at 6 a.m. Really, throwing a party on top of full-time caring is quite an ask, but where you're concerned, I seem to be able to find unexpected reserves of strength, even though I'm running on empty.

The garden is pristine. Festoon lights are up all around the garden. Wine and beers have taken over the fridges. Furniture has been moved and rugs rolled up. Canapés are made, with more being donated by friends. Ice is bought. Helpers are briefed. The fire pit is ready. Outside, chill-out areas have been decorated with blankets and cushions.

You roll down the corridor fifteen minutes before kick-off. You are calm, silent. You speak through music and put on Ryan Adams's 'La Cienega Just Smiled' – possibly to calm me or even lift me, or to say I love you and thank you for this party. You know I love that song – an early memory of our time together.

Our guests arrive on time. By chance my brother Graham is over from Australia and has just this morning landed back from a trip to Kenya. My sister Fiona pops down from Shropshire too. Thank heavens for my siblings leaning in. I go and squeeze into my black cord boiler suit and rock-chick boots. I put on red lipstick to make me feel more energised, and lashings of black mascara. It makes a change from leggings, trainers and a blank visage.

I panic. The room is suddenly very full and loud. There were so many more people I wanted to invite but we had to stay contained. About fifty-five are here. Roddy, ex-army, booms out for the room to be quiet. You wheel yourself out of your disco corner and make a small speech, starting by excusing the cannula but it gives you a constant supply of cocaine for the evening. That goes down well. You talk about it being fifty-eight years since you started DJing at the Bali Hai Bar at the Locarno Ballroom in Birmingham. You thank Helen Thomas, your boss from Radio 2, for coming. You credit yourself for bringing her to the station from Radio 4 to be your *Drivetime* producer (she doesn't argue this point). You also thank Mark Goodier. Then you play your first track, the same one you started with at the Bali Hai: the Four Tops 'Can't Help My Self' … Purple, green and red from the disco light shimmer over the walls and vaulted ceiling. Tacky but suitable.

The dancing starts. It's a slow start, as there's a lot of eating, drinking and talking going on, but soon my girl-friends are giving their legs a great workout. I realise that the main room of our house is made for a party like this. Every bit of its thirty-three-feet length is being used.

Your boss Helen works the room brilliantly. She gets plugged by a songwriter friend about his new single, but mainly she gets lots of praise for hiring Vernon Kay and delights in showing me a video of him tossing the caber in Bute. I ask if she was there. She said she couldn't go there *and* make our party. She chose you, Johnnie. Her devotion and loyalty to you is extraordinary.

Mark Goodier steps in to DJ so you can go and smoke. That's as bad as you get – clearly music and survival are your mindset, in the end; not drugs. But then you have always, since I've known you, been a pro. And you probably only said it to wind me up. You have one G&T and otherwise it's water and popcorn that sustains you. It's sort of odd. You sit in your wheelchair with your iPad next to your valve amp and oxygen machine, and there you stay. You don't want to mingle, though of course you are a sitting duck for people to come and have one-on-one chats. They need that. Many have not seen you all year. This is their goodbye, though I don't think you twig that. I realise as I talk to our guests that you are delighted not to have to make small talk around the room. And then I think back to all our supper parties where you have played music at the end. It dawns on me – this was to get you out of talking! You are a radio man. You have always enjoyed being in a studio alone. A one-way conversation. Because, honestly, you're not very interested in people. It's the music, man! That is your motivation and this is the perfect style of party for you now. It doesn't mean you haven't partied well in the past, because you have. From our wedding party and your book launch after-party at the Union Club, to Bob Harris's unforgettable sixtieth birthday or the balls at Goodwood, you've danced, laughed, drunk and revelled.

There's excitement from anyone who gets their track played. All I asked for was Sister Sledge's 'We Are Family'. I dance with my siblings and think to myself that I never, ever thought that the four of us would dance together while you DJed. And yet here we are – my high point of the evening. I see you smile; you love me dancing. The rock-chick boots soon get replaced by trainers.

Gorgeous Poshie, one of our dear, more ethereal friends who has made you so many cakes, soups and goodies in your periods of ill health that she named herself 'Soup Pest', comes up to me and says how brilliant this is. That we would all be at your funeral, but this way we can all celebrate you while you're here. And that's it, Johnnie. While you just wanted to see people dancing to the music you play one more time, we are actually providing something far deeper and more profound for our friends.

The music ends at 11 p.m. You announce that this is the final song you will ever live DJ. You *stun* the room by putting on a slow one: 'The Rose' by Bette Midler. 'But,

Johnnie, we need a banger to end on!' I shout across the room. I apologise later for my outburst. The music is your area, and you want to end on a slow dance because in your day that's what you did. We all adjust and grab someone to dance with. Our friend Martyn grabs me, and we sing our hearts out to a song that I got you to love. So in a way I am flattered. There's a huge cheer for you at the end. 'Hip-hip-hooray!' we all chant. And within minutes, like one of the Rolling Stones leaving the stadium quicker than Jumpin' Jack Flash, you're rolling out of there, waving from your wheelchair and heading down the corridor. It is the last time most people in the room will see you. Some leave, though a hardcore stay on. Honestly, no one there will ever forget their farewell evening to you, and while you didn't talk that much, they don't mind because they understand the man you are. A DJ.

You fall on your bed, which makes undressing you hard. Your feet and legs are cold. You are shattered. I tuck you in, forgetting half the things I should do. You are worried. I am worried. Although I don't share that; I just tell you that you were brilliant and that I love you. I return to the party in need of red wine. Gradually guests leave and I clear up till 2 a.m., only to be woken at 4.45 a.m. by the cockerel next door.

Four people stay the night. In the morning, they help me move the furniture back. I leave you in bed. I am too scared that you will have popped off from the strain, so I wait till they have all gone, because if you have I know I want to be alone with you. I am so afraid that I wait to take you a tea until 10.45 a.m. My heart is in my mouth, but there you are, eyes open. And you stay there for the day while I clear up the trash, take down the lights and rearrange everything. I finish around 5 p.m. and slump.

It took four intense, long days of my life to set up the party and then clear it up. There was hardly a piece of furniture that wasn't moved, an area that wasn't lit up. I did food and booze galore and mixed with all our friends. By the end of it I am exhausted, and for me it would have been worth all that energy if you had seemed a little more grateful. You honestly don't seem to have enjoyed yourself. Our guests did – they had a great time – but you can't even thank me with sincerity in your voice or heart. It was too much for you, but specifically people coming to talk to you. You wished you'd been unreachable up on a stage and could have just played music. That was all you wanted – to check you still had the power to make people dance. It wasn't about socialising with people. I don't regret it one bit. It's amazing that we threw a party with you in your state, really amazing, and the thank-yous flood in, but I wonder if you are just too far gone with your health now to actually enjoy yourself.

The next day my body has spoken. I sleep all morning, as do you. The DJing has taken its toll, and so has the hostessing. Never again, Johnnie. I am NOT doing another party for you! But somehow, I don't think you'll be asking me to.

I am smiling to myself here. You obviously forgot that today is *Rock Show* recording day. I've just heard you putting on your voice. And I know you're in your PJs having leapt out of bed when Liz texted you. How can you pull that out of the hat still? If only you could help with the practical stuff too. I am secretly bloody smug that for once I am in bed and you are working.

You have been telling me for months that you only have three weeks left. I've stopped taking it seriously as it has been doing me in. However, a week after the party you are still struggling. There's been a lot of black humour passed among our friends that if the party didn't finish you off, what the hell will? Maybe the after-effects. I give you a bath today (I actually think I'm good at it, and you agree with me). It's an intimate time and you often share more personal thoughts then. You say that you've gone downhill in the past few days. You say that even moving your position in bed can make you out of breath. And you are pretty much on Level 9 of oxygen all the time now – the highest level. I know you are being truthful, as when you swing your legs out of the bath (from the lift), you don't have the strength to stand up for me to put your dressing gown on. For the first time ever you say, 'I hope I die soon.'

I am being given therapy. With my therapist Martine I cry for the first time this year about the fact that I will lose you. Until now I've been in control. What a relief to know I care. She sees that I'm holding on, keeping it all together. She's delighted that I cry. We talk about you a lot. In a way she is preparing me for grief. We talk about your wildness and my lack of it; that I recognised in you an animal I wish I was, and you recognised in me one who could keep you on the straight and narrow. But have I been just too straight with you? I know that behind my back you're a monkey, having a puff and goodness knows what else when you can, trying to break the rules without me knowing. It's my role to be the strict one because if I give you an inch, you take a mile.

I'm in London to check on the flat – which didn't sell, and I am secretly very happy about it. I don't want to lose this connection to the city. I take an early-morning walk through Primrose Hill park up to the classic view of London. I choke up. My heart immediately feels heavy without Darcey Dog at my side, and knowing you will never see this glorious view again – the city in which you lived for most of your life, looking magnificent on this hazy, late-summer morning. I realise I really am already grieving: you, me and Darcey. That was our true inner family, and soon I will be the only one left. Tears start to tumble.

I have two meetings and then I can't wait to return to you. I have your beloved sourdough bread from Little Bread Pedlar on board – possibly your final taste of London.

I lie in bed knowing that I am flying to Rome for two days in the morning. I need to have some meetings with possible heads of department for the film. In February when I went to Sardinia I was overwhelmed with emotion and fear. In

July when I went to France I felt confident you would be there on my return. Now, I am quite calm, because I am OK for you to go. I don't want you suffering any more than you have to. I silently speak to the cells of your body, telling them that I am fine for you to go. I give you permission. You can stop fretting for me. With all my soul I pass that message into your cells.

You get up early to wave me off. You want no one to go in to see you today. The fridge is stacked. You are happy to be on your own. I think about animals and how they like to be alone when they die and wonder if that is what fate has stored up. Much of me thinks you will choose to go when I'm not there, either today or in the future. And I don't mind. In fact, it would be a relief to always remember you alive, with that spark you have.

I return from Rome full of excitement – as ever after a break. The meetings were all a success. I love that feeling of being alive and creative, making bonds with others, and together we will make something special.

You, on the other hand, have taken up smoking like there's no tomorrow. Since we agreed you could smoke at your party, you are now doing so as a matter of course during the day and before bed. You once told me smoking is a socially acceptable form of suicide, and maybe this is what it's about, but I also know that the smell of smoke makes my stomach heave. I am, as I've always told you, allergic to cigarette smoke. That was discovered when I was thirty. So having you wheel down the corridor reeking of it is such a repulsion that I cannot come and help you get into bed or kiss you goodnight. Not for the first time, I think to myself, *It's the fags or me. You choose which you want.* But you know – and so do I – that you will have both. I can hardly demand exclusivity at this point in your life.

I dream that you are driving me to Primrose Hill. You are dressed as you used to be – a shirt, a jacket, good jeans. You don't have any oxygen machine on you. You seem a good ten years younger. You are fit and the Johnnie you used to be, and honestly, when I wake I think you must have died as the dream was so real. To be reminded of how our life was really hurts. It reminds me of how shrunken it has become.

This week we 'celebrated' twenty-three years of meeting. We are both tired and down. It is an awful evening, despite me serving lovely food and wine. You call it a negative night. My fatigue is getting deeper and deeper. I'm aching to return to my power and yet you show no sign of letting me do so.

Self-preservation is becoming my main concern. The words 'care home' are now entering our vocabulary, because I don't know how much more I can take. We discuss you 'releasing me' from caring in November. It sounds cruel, and it's not what I wanted. I want you to die in our home, but I am almost breaking with the effort of it all. As I said on our anniversary … I've really had it with the noisy oxygen machines and long oxygen tubing, pee bottles and commodes, wheelchairs, the constant making of meals, laundry and getting you dressed. The only thing I am not sick of is giving you a bath.

I see your self-destruct button is rearing its head. Your smoking reaches new levels. You are lost in a world of your phone and iPad. I've no idea what you're reading or looking at; you have become too closed to share. It's hard to get through to you. I guess you want to feel alive, and yet the sadness of the smoking is that it's indicative of you giving up.

I have let Helen Thomas at Radio 2 know that you will stop broadcasting at the end of October. She is sad but, like me, she's glad it's your decision and that you can have a proper send-off. You have a chance to play all your favourite tracks one last time, and receive the love. With Helen – and Sharon, the head PR at Radio 2 – we will plan the announcement and press release. There'll be more attention, of course – as if we need that. Do you crave quiet and privacy as much as I do? We still haven't opened all the cards you've been sent. It's like your cancer time all over again. The love that is sent is beautiful, but energy has to be found to deal with it.

The discussion about a care home is firming up. Rather than leaving it as a concept, I'm doing research. You have reached a place where you want me to be free, and while I struggle with the thought of you being incarcerated, I too want me to be free – at least next year. Here's my dilemma: *ANTONIA*, my passion-piece film, has been delayed and delayed because of you. And because I'm not just the writer, and second producer, but also currently attached as the director, it will be all-consuming. It does not mix with caring. Our team have all accepted the delay from this year, but we can't really expect them to go on and on waiting, especially Jayne-Ann who, as lead producer, has been breaking her balls to make this manifest. If by chance you are still around in January, you will be sleeping most of the time, with bedpans your major need. I am not doing that. I wouldn't be strong enough.

Of course, I do wonder if you stopping the show will take away your remaining power. Your life's purpose will be over. But what I am learning is that the human spirit – especially yours – knows no bounds of strength. How are you even alive now, with the dreadful state of your lungs?

I've had the conversation with Helen about your replacements on the shows. It seems Bob Harris was right; he is the natural successor to *Sounds of the 70s*. Shaun Keaveny will do the *Rock Show*. I know you told Helen I should do *Sounds of the 70s*, but that would *never* have happened. I'm sure she laughed as you suggested it, but then you always have been my biggest radio fan. I told her that Liz 'Queen of Rock' Barnes should be considered for the *Rock Show*. Helen knows her mind and she's gone for safe, reliable choices, and thank goodness they are both real radio men and not 'celebs'. I'm not sure if I'll be able to listen to them, though. Having the conversation was hard. To realise that you really are stopping, that it's the end of an era, a career, a lifetime of radio – my heart sinks at the thought. I can't imagine what your heart is doing as you approach your final shows. You will announce it on Sunday, 6 October. How I dread the attention. How many texts and emails will I have to respond to? I'd better leave a day clear to deal with them.

I have great gratitude for your chariot – I know you love pottering around on it. For a man who has always loved vehicles, I give praise for the small joy that (almost) to the end you will enjoy driving something. After it's had a service, I need to drive it back to your room. Holy schmoly, that thing shoots down the corridor with such speed I scream out loud and think I'm going to crash. I swear it could go 30mph. You laugh. The servicing man has left it in fifth gear, while you keep it in first. This begs a question – who needs FIVE gears in a wheelchair?

I see a noticeable change in you. Dark rings have formed around your eyes – it's beyond bags; it's the look of an old person. And without doubt you are spending more time in bed than out. You've also stopped using your beloved blue velvet chair. For the time you spend in the main room 'up', you are staying in the wheelchair. I can't remember when you last got out of pyjamas. Your appetite still exists – but mainly for carbs and comfort food. On Friday evening, which is becoming our date night, you eat almost nothing of the sea trout, samphire, spinach and chickpea dinner that I've lovingly served, but boy, after I've removed the offending healthy food, do you go for some manchego and fruity cheese biscuits, cantucinni biscuits dipped in dessert wine and then an ENTIRE large bag of sweet and salty popcorn!

You have suggested cutting your steroids back from four a day to three, and Rohan Mehta, your consultant, is very much of the opinion that you are the one who knows the right level. Steroids lead to the munchies, and you feel that eating less rubbish may be good for you. Or perhaps you just want to reduce this way of propping up your strength. You take so many pills to keep you going, but more and more I realise that is not what you want. Indeed, I feel quite keenly that while we are not there yet, the dreaded moment may come in November or early December, once you have stopped broadcasting. And let me be quite honest, I hope that is the case. It sounds harsh, but it's nearly the moment to call time.

Your son Sam calls to see how I am. I love that he's concerned about me as well as you. How I wish he lived here and not in Australia. I'm on my early-morning Saturday drive up to Shaftesbury to get your croissant. Somehow this amuses him. He has heard that we're discussing the idea of a care home for you. I hear my voice crack. I cannot hide my emotion of how bloody hard it has been for me this year, how unbelievably challenging you can be to manage. Sam knows you, and he gets it. He laughs when I tell him you are pathologically programmed to be bad. He realises for the first time the incredible toll this is taking on me. I don't mean for him to know this, but it splurges out. I tell him I know no one who has sacrificed as much as I have this year, looking after you. Sam is completely understanding. I thank him for being just one of four people in your family who regularly keep in touch with me to see how I'm doing. Your nieces Michelle and Trudi and cousin Mal are the other three. I love them for recognising how tough this time is and what it is doing to me.

Sam doesn't know if he should come over now or wait for the funeral. I suggest the latter as you two have said your physical goodbye at Heathrow last November. You agree with this completely and even say he shouldn't bother with the funeral. I inwardly disagree on that, as I think Beth will need his brotherly support.

As for care homes, I have suggested that for November you must be here at home. I will need to protect you from your own fallout after stopping work. I think it will hit you hard and that will be one of the most important times for me to support you. To put you into a home just before Christmas feels utterly churlish and wrong, so we have agreed that looking at January onwards would be a good idea. You tell Sam it's what you want because you think it might be fun (really?!), but mainly you want to free me after such an intensive year. I think we both know that it won't happen, though. I'm pretty sure you will call time before that, so possibly it's just an emotional crutch to help keep me going. The thought of light at the end of a long, dark, claustrophobic tunnel.

Insomnia is raising its head again. I'm listening out for you, getting woken by the smallest sound. And in those hours when I toss and turn, any time between 1 a.m. and 6 a.m., I find myself dwelling on the eulogy you want me to do. I've thought of so many openings, so many lines, so many angles. I can only say what I believe, and there will be much that I must not say. I mean, honestly, darling, is it really wise for any man to ask his wife to do this hugely important sign-off? It's just too tempting to complain about all your faults. But of course, you trust me, as you should. You know that despite your multiple flaws, no one has ever fought your corner as hard as I have. Unless you have upset me – and then you feel the full force of my rage, as you should. But how on earth do I sum up someone like you?

I'm out of control. I'm like a spider trying to avoid getting sucked down the plughole but the water is speeding up and I can't hold on. A force is happening beyond my control. I know you are getting worse and suddenly there's not enough time to look after you, get everything done, stay on top of things. I took a sleeping pill last night and still woke four times. I think I hear you ringing a bell, so I get up and find you fast asleep. We keep having power cuts, which make your machine beep constantly and the phone make a weird sound when it comes back on. Thus, I'm oversleeping, not getting enough time to prep everything before I go to an early-morning class. I rush in to your room with your early tea and breakfast on one tray, telling you I can't stop as I'm behind schedule. I fling open your curtains, wheel out the Alien, but I leave the pee bottle full and you gawping, 'Where are you going?' Yoga! Tennis! Fitness class! Back later! Should I be cancelling these classes? I'm starting to feel guilty and yet they keep me going.

My body is out of control too. I am certain the sertraline has filled out my entire stomach area. Or is it comfort eating? Clothes that hung on me last year now fit like a tight girdle. It's so depressing. I know we're all supposed to be body positive, but when my midriff stops certain yoga poses because it's too large, I can't help feeling ashamed. Dare I stop the antidepressants? Will I crumble again as I did in January? Or am I now a hardened carer who has already done so much grieving for our life that I'll be fine? Do I register with a nutritionist? Do I wait till after your final curtain has fallen? I need to be on top of me, my life. Being out of control is my worst state, but to your credit, when I get like this you are supportive, even though you are the cause. You put your own dilemma to one side and focus on mine. When I can get you out of your bubble you are the most wonderful advisor – still.

It doesn't help that I'm filming a short film in two weeks – a directorial debut. I'm paying for it, so I'm asking favours from lots of lovely crew and actors. People are being so kind. They love the script. I feel love all around. I just need more sleep and time.

Helen the vicar has offered to come and give us Communion again on Saturday. She will be our only visitor that day. Two things she prays for strike us: 'That Johnnie will live as long as possible' and 'Forgive us our sins.' When I see Helen out I return to you, and I'm laughing. So are you. 'Bet you didn't pray for me to live as long as possible!' you quip. No, I bloody didn't! Honestly, Johnnie, our humour … Then you add, 'You don't have any sins to forgive, unlike me.' Really, Duke, I'm not perfect. I have sins just like everyone. Just not as many or as large as yours!

I make an enormous social-media mistake afterwards. I am so taken by the prettiness of Helen's travelling Communion kit that I put up an Insta post of it. The floodgates open with friends getting in touch: 'Tiggy! Is Johnnie OK?' It's as if I've said it was your FINAL Communion. We're not there yet.

TRIP THE LIGHT FANTASTIC

The *Rock Show* got rescheduled to 11 p.m. on a Friday night. This didn't affect you as, since Covid, these were all done as pre-records with your Queen of Rock producer Liz Barnes. While I don't have a great knowledge of or affinity for rock music, I have at times listened alone in my bedroom at 11 p.m. while you already slept in your own room with your oxygen concentrator at your side. It's hard to comprehend that the man I see struggling with breath on a daily basis is pumping out these songs with such energy.

The one band you seem to champion a lot is Greta Van Fleet, and – spoiler alert – I discover it's not a woman, but a band of blokes. I love the title of their song 'Trip the Light Fantastic', so I'm borrowing it, as I believe I tripped the light fantastic myself when I did something with extraordinary foresight in September 2023. I was having my nails painted one Saturday morning and had the most overwhelming sense that I should text Sam in Australia. Sam and I have always got on well. I've never tried to be a stepmother to either of your children. Why would I? For a start my age is directly between yours and theirs, and they were both fully formed adults when we met. In Sam's case, he has been a wonderful addition to my life and I will always be there for him and his family. There was a plan that he would come over the following April, in 2024, for a visit. However, without telling you, I texted him to say that my hunch was that he should come over this autumn. I felt it was too risky to wait till the spring.

He trusted my instinct and booked to come in November for ten days – and what a wonderful ten days it was. We had Sunday lunch at the Grosvenor Arms in Hindon, sitting by the roaring fire. He came with us on a hospital visit for an ultrasound on your heart, and we then went to the Beckford Arms for lunch. And possibly best of all, I booked the two of you into the Pig at Combe as I really wanted you to have a small road trip and some boys' time together. Unlike you, Sam is a foodie, and there he could try the delights of the wood-fired oven in the garden folly and their twenty-five-mile menu for supper. The next day you drove on to the coast to meet up with Beth for fish and chips at the Hive Beach Café at Burton Bradstock. You and your offspring all together. I knew it would be the last time that would happen and suggested you got some great photos of the three of you. I didn't mean a couple of badly taken selfies, but never mind. It's a day that will remain with the three of you forever.

For Sam's final weekend you took him for breakfast at Guy Ritchie's Compton Abbas Airfield so you could eat while you watched small planes take off and land. Sam used to have a flying licence and it's just the boys' sort of thing that excites you. But perhaps the finest afternoon of the stay was when d'Arcy and Gary invited us to Sunday lunch along with our other besties, Jane and Charles. The gang of six plus one. None of them had ever met Sam and they wanted to do this for you. How they loved him. And how surprised they were that he is the absolute antithesis of you. They were thinking, how did such a normal, balanced, intelligent man come from your loins? To quote Sam's best ever line: 'I grew up surrounded by sex, drugs and rock 'n' roll, but I rebelled by getting a degree and going into banking.' I watched you glow with pride at their obvious affection and admiration for him. Somewhere towards the end of lunch, Charles, an imposing man who works in the City, leaned over to Sam and told him not to worry about a thing; they would all be there to help look after his dad.

You drove Sam to the airport the next day. You had it all planned. Your best 007 Seiko watch which you had won at a silent auction for Salisbury District Hospital Stars Appeal, was in your pocket. You knew this would be your physical goodbye. The only thing you inherited from your father was a watch, and so you wanted both Sam and Beth to have a watch from your own collection of wristwear. Handing it over to Sam was a poignant moment for you both and it was the culmination of an amazing ten days. (After you die, I hand Beth the small Seiko and indeed most of your remaining watch collection.)

Sam says he will be indebted to me for the rest of his life for getting him over when I did – when you could still walk, drive and enjoy life. It was a treasured time that really did trip the light fantastic – whatever that actually means.

THE FINAL SHOW

It's a big build-up to the announcement: press releases, social-media posts – all to be approved by us. The network approaches it all with huge respect. When you record it on your regular Wednesday-afternoon slot I take in a coffee and ask if it's done – the announcement. It is, and yet both you and Liz are so nonchalant about it. No big drama or emotion. You just pop it in at the end of an email about someone else's dad dying of pulmonary fibrosis. Oh, yes – I'll be stopping in a few weeks. Throw-away. So you.

Boom. Sunday, 6 October 2024 at 3.54 p.m., your listeners hear that you are stopping. As your publicist (among many of my jobs), I post an Insta of you waving goodbye in your old Wogan House studio. Beautiful messages are left under this, and what I love is that they all get it. They love you, but they know you're sick and everyone wishes you well. My tweet is a photo of you and Bob Harris at the Eagles concert in Hyde Park in 2022. Robert Plant is singing on the huge screen behind you: 'From one friend to another.' Bob texts me, delighted that I posted a message of such public support of him taking over.

The Radio 2 PR team ask about all the interview requests. We turn them all down, even the *Radio Times* (who, let's face it, have never put you on the cover and so haven't really earned any brownie points from us, despite the radio legend you are supposed to be). I tell them you are doing NO MORE INTERVIEWS. Then Rebecca Hardy from the *Mail* texts me. She has done two articles on us before: after your cancer and after mine. No, I tell her. Then she says how about she comes down and interviews just me? You and I discuss this and agree that would be OK. Then she mentions having ten minutes with you. She's bloody clever!

You're still in bed when she arrives. She and I talk, and it's such a delicate balance, treading the line between the fact that I love you and will miss you, and the fact that I feel bloody tired and trapped, and struggle being your full-time carer. I check on you, and before long you wheel yourself in with your opening gambit to Rebecca: 'She can't wait for me to die!!' It's so funny and magically you set the tone for your interview. We laugh all the way through, which is the very last thing she expected when we were going to be discussing your demise.

Murray, the photographer, arrives – this is the fourth time he's snapped us. Again, like Rebecca, the first time was after your cancer in our Marylebone flat. They have both been the press-media constants of our life, so somehow it feels totally right that they are here in yet another of our homes. Murray is a fan; he's so thrilled to be with us that he can't stop talking. You are fantastically open and friendly. I end up making everyone a sandwich because it's gone 2 p.m. and we haven't even taken a shot yet; it's just banter and laughter, and a bit of hair and make-up. You are talking too much. I remind the room that you're recording your show at 2.30 p.m. and must conserve your energy. I need to conserve mine too. I'm so tired by the time the photos start that I find it hard to muster a smile. You keep delaying the start of your show. You only have three more left. They are so precious and all have to be as good as possible. It's 4.30 p.m. before you get going. Before the recording starts you wheel down the corridor to your den and start listening to tracks. The music drifts up to the kitchen. I walk in to find Murray having a moment; he is not just moved, he's emotional. 'That track …' He excuses himself. I know that it's more than the track. It reminds me of the huge connection there is between you and your listeners. I forget that sometimes; maybe I'm even blind to it. I know it exists because of all the messages, cards and emails that keep arriving, but with Murray I can actually SEE it. He doesn't realise that in that moment he is giving me the understanding of what thousands of people think about you and how very deep their feelings go.

The *Mail* team are with us for well over five hours. I am done for at the end, and worried about you having enough energy for your show, and while your voice sounds croaky at the start, you dig, dig, dig deep and you astound me when I overhear some links. As ever I wonder how you do it. You tell me later that you have to dig down here – you hold your fist to your solar plexus, the seat of strength. You don't do that for me. Just your shows. I get it.

The article is out in the Saturday *Mail*. In the photo you look incredibly happy, spoilt almost. I look pale and tired; I'm hardly smiling. As a result of that article more cards arrive. At least 100 to Johnnie Walker DJ, Dorset. I have to applaud the Post Office; this is a good PR story for them. The reaction to the article is good. It prompts a few more people to get in touch who want to visit (or possibly it's a coincidence). The list is currently Hugh Bonneville (Thursday), which will be hilarious, I know, and just what we need. Then on the wait list is Robert Plant, Michael Eavis, Richard Allinson and your fellow pirate on Radio England Roger 'Twiggy' Day. I need to get through my film shoot and your final show before booking them in.

My shoot is a triumph – I can now legitimately call myself a director. You're thrilled for me and have been incredibly good at keeping your head down and being undemanding. Thank you. I dig as deep as you do for a show, with the result that this weekend I want complete solitude to recoup my energy and do all those things I should, like clean the commode from head to toe and defrost the freezer. Sometimes mundane domesticity is just what the soul needs. I've also caught up on death-facing admin. We've checked your will, done your letter of wishes, contacted the bank, stuck your DNR (do not resuscitate) in an envelope on the front door in the event that paramedics are called out when I'm not here. It all has to be done. The last thing I want is any strife after you've gone.

You sleep and sleep. It's what Nurse Emma said you would do, and she was right. In one week your final show will go out. Friends ask if you're sad, and I tell them relief is all you feel. We both do.

The last song: that's what everyone wants to know about. The *Mail*; Helen your boss. The coolest person about it is Liz, your producer. She knows that you'll find the right thing. You've been toying with the Royal Scots Dragoon Guards playing 'Amazing Grace' – one of those freak Number Ones that happened in the Seventies. 'You can't go out on f***ing bagpipes,' I say in my usual forthright manner. 'I mean, you're not Scottish and you hate the bagpipes …'

I'm at my weekly yoga class, and as I stand in Mountain Pose it comes to me: Judy Collins's 'Amazing Grace'. Back at home I bring my computer, along with your sourdough toast and coffee, into your bedroom. I sit on the lovely wingback chair, as you want to dictate your song list. I throw out the idea of Judy Collins and you tell me that you too had thought that and had just listened to it. It goes on the list as the one to beat. I suggest it will have everyone crying, which is just what you want, and I could use it at your funeral too, so there's a tie-in. Honestly, the things I think about – and voice.

You are itching to dictate your list for the show – the songs spill out of you quicker than I can type. Mink DeVille. The Staple Singers. Johnny Nash. I question why these, and you say simply because you love them – and I never knew. Sister Sledge's 'We Are Family' you want because that's how you look upon your listeners. Elton and Kiki are a given, as is Lou Reed's 'Walk on the Wild Side' because Liz has pulled out that great clip where he realises you are the man that made his career in Europe. You suddenly interject, 'Have you thought that I might pop off after the last show?' I cough, wipe away some tears and say we need to get the list done. (Yes, of course I have thought that, but it's just too close and soon to contemplate that happening.) Songs go in and come out. In the space of twenty minutes there are far too many on the list. You have three punk songs, which I suggest is two too many, and you agree as we have to edit the choices down quite a bit. After a day of reviewing your choices, you go into the show with this list:

HOUR ONE

George Harrison – What is Life
Sister Sledge – We are Family
Roger Daltrey – Giving it All Away
Elton John And Kiki Dee – Don't Go Breaking My Heart
Rod Stewart– Mandolin Wind
Neil Diamond – Holly Holy
Peter Gabriel – Solsbury Hill

The Rolling Stones – Wild Horses/Dead Flowers
Jackson Browne – Fountain of Sorrow
Stevie Wonder – He's Misstra Know-it-All
Mink Deville – Spanish Stroll
Simon & Garfunkel – Song for the Asking

HOUR TWO

Bob Seger – Main Street
Cat Stevens – Father and Son
Nils Lofgren – Shine Silently
Staple Singers – If You're Ready
David Bowie – Drive-in Saturday
Lou Reed – Walk on the Wild Side
Skids – Into the Valley
Van Morrison – Into the Mystic
Paul McCartney & Wings – Band on the Run
Judy Collins – Amazing Grace

Needless to say, it becomes very organic during the show – some songs change and a lot move, often because of trails and timings, and often because you change your mind because a song is too long.

Liz and Paul come down for the final recording. Paul insists it is the right thing to do; he knows you shouldn't end your career by shutting your laptop alone in your den. I get up early to make soda bread, prepare a lunch, clean the floors, get you bathed and dressed. (What? No PJs today?!) Flowers arrive from Helen and Laura at Radio 2 – stunning autumnal colours, and for the first time today I cry. I rush to get a vase and put them in your den for the show. I print out the final song list as Paul and Liz's taxi pulls up in the drive.

It's funny to have their injection of energy in the house, but it's a good thing. They bring flowers, a candle, Bombay Sapphire and a special bottle of Jameson whiskey for you (a new addition to your morning coffee, to go with the first two fags of the day. I learn that Irish whiskey is softer than Scottish so for you it's a delicious addition to your first brew). Plus, an audio surprise: a recording of Sir Rod Stewart making a wonderful impromptu tribute to you, which is to be dropped into the show. My second tears of the day fall.

We prep your den, ring your friend Rodney for an emergency extra microphone for me, and have lunch. I'm already quite tired by the time we start the show at about 3 p.m. You want me on it and to sit opposite you all the way through, until the final half-hour when you want to be alone.

With the four of us in your den it's quite cosy. You don't tell me anything about what you want me to say. That's because you don't know; you don't have a single note in front of you except the list of former producers to thank and the song choices. The rest of it is all off the cuff. Throughout, I am on the backfoot and completely surprised when you suddenly look at me and ask something. 'Do you shine silently?' you ask after Nils Lofgren's song. I have no idea what you're on about. 'I do it noisily,' I respond in a panic, and you laugh, and laugh. It's like that all the way through: I'm a stunned rabbit and come out with garbage. I keep surprising you with the things I say. I find myself talking about my mother, how she hates music and never wanted radios in the car. Why am I talking about her on the radio? She is such a good, kind, Christian woman, and at ninety-three, the most enquiring, fascinated person in the family. I think it's because she is the antithesis of me. Yet I was so influenced by her. I've always fought against that influence. I clearly need therapy about her, but not on-air. (I will later wake in the middle of the night and regret most of the things I said, but I will not share this with you or your production team, as the show is about you, not me. I was only there as a foil to set you off in different directions. But I really do worry that people will think, 'Shut up, Tiggy. It's his last show.' And if they do, I will not blame them. I agree!)

There is one thing I am pleased about: I tell you on-air how proud I am that you have carried on broadcasting these past ten months (which I've not said enough privately). I alone have seen the struggle and the great depths you have had to mine. My voice croaks very slightly. You seem touched and thank me.

For the final half-hour, Liz sets up her computer in our living room and FaceTimes you from the other end of the house, so that you can be completely alone with your listeners, and not distracted by us. She, Paul and I listen to your final links together.

And I cry for the third time today.

There is champagne, photos, and then suddenly Liz and Paul's taxi arrives. Your final show is in the can. You look at me across our dining-room table where we sit, exhausted, and say, 'I think it's just hit me.' And I think it has.

You eat very little supper and are in bed by 8 p.m. I sit on the edge of your bed and tell you how proud I am of you. And I am. You have been an incredible broadcaster for so many years. You are the best, I tell you – unique – and will be so missed.

And now my anxiety starts that you may now stop. Some force has kept you going all year; you have outlasted any doctor's predictions and I believe it is radio that has been your secret weapon. That weapon has now been put down. You have surrendered to your illness. I really do worry that all of a sudden you won't be there, which is probably the reason that I wake at 4 a.m. and start writing.

I continue to wake at 4 a.m. night after night, and every morning I am more aware that I may walk in to find your body rigid. There is no doubt, the exhaustion has hit you, and now, a week after the show went out, I am more worried than ever that you are slowing down. You have pretty much migrated to bed except for supper and an hour of TV most evenings.

Has the force that has kept you alive ended?

Let's talk about that last show, though, because I tell you, my love, it was a masterclass in how to bow out. You were upset that Bob Seger, Van Morrison and Wings were cut, but it was more important to get the talk in. You and Sally, Rod's lovely clip, your stories – it was just perfect. As for your last words: *So thank you for being with me all these years. Take good care of yourself and those you love. And may we walk into the future with our heads held high and happiness in our hearts. God bless you …* They could not have been better said. You never use a script; the words just come, and they were perfect. Us listening to the show go out with no one else around was the perfect thing. When Judy Collins sang 'Amazing Grace', I sat opposite you and we held both our hands together, tears running down my face, tears in your eyes. It was one of the best moments of eye contact we've ever had. It was a huge, profound moment for you, for me, for your myriad listeners.

The day after the show airs I am euphoric. You have glowing reviews in *The Telegraph* and the *Daily Mail,* and the social-media posts and comments are off the scale. The feedback from the radio world is simply superb. You nailed it. But it's not just pride that I feel, it is that an inordinate weight has lifted from my shoulders. It hits me how, for twenty-three years, we have almost never been off-duty. What if a popstar dies? What if someone wants you for an interview? Are you free for this event? Will you sign this photo? Please listen to my CD! What if you did or said something that got you cancelled? Well, now it's all over. The public life. If Mick Jagger or Paul McCartney should suddenly keel over, you don't need to respond. For the first time ever we can be a private couple. Normal. Just getting through your illness in our own way. The only sense that you were once a public figure is that each day more and more cards find their way to us – on average twenty a day. And the beauty is that because you are in bed all day, you have the time to read them. You cannot believe the things people write, how much you have meant to them. You are the friend they never met, so incredibly important in their lives, and in a way they are grieving you. For many it is the end of their line with Radio 2, and I cannot help but think how very much the BBC undervalued you. There's no point in getting upset, but you always said how they didn't realise just what they had in you. I suspect when they look at the final show's listening figures and see the media coverage, they will realise. I know I am biased, but who else has that special connection that you do with your listeners? You had a God-given communication talent.

It's early November and Quincy Jones has just died. We do not have to react; we can just hear the reactions of others. Meanwhile the cards continue to flow in. There are hundreds and hundreds now, and I've run out of shelf space. Two lovely letters arrive as well. Michael Palin sends such a personal, kind message, telling you that your show was his deceased wife Helen's favourite radio show and how he listened to the final one thinking of her. And TIM DAVIE – only the director general of the BBC! You probably think he's never heard of you, but his letter is so warm, so congrat-ulatory, so appreciative of how you have worked through your illness. He talks of your dedication to music and your listeners. He's even heard our caring podcast – he mentions ME! Fancy us being on his radar. It's humbling. We both say the same thing, as we so often do: it deserves to be framed. It's now in the loo. Because you are touched, you send him a thank-you card. Still a gentleman, Johnnie. (Months later I will meet Tim Davie and he will tell me that while he is sent many cards, yours is one of the only ones he has kept.)

I ask you if you're sure you quit at the right time. You are. Utterly. You didn't have another show in you. And I know you mean it. Timing has always been your forte.

LA DOLCE VITA

The moment I would like to live again is our first kiss, but the evening I would love to recreate is the best one we ever shared. If ever there was a movie about you, this would be my favourite scene. And I know it would be yours too, for in our whirlwind life, this evening alone stood out as a moment of perfection.

In September 2005 we were driving back from the Italian Formula 1 race at Monza – the one where I ran after Kimi Räikkönen in the paddock (he was my favourite driver; the feeling was clearly not mutual, though, and he got away from me). As we started our meandering drive back home, you behind the wheel of your latest impulse purchase – a burgundy Mercedes sports car (which had 'spoken to you' as you drove past the showroom – honestly!) – and me clutching the map and the *Michelin Guide* the way I loved to do as chief navigator, I suggested a quick detour to the beautiful harbour of Portofino – possibly the only 'fishing' village in Europe where the shops edging it are Prada and Gucci. I don't imagine a single one of the beautiful boats bobbing on the water belong to fishermen. It is picturesque beyond belief, and very hard to negotiate in a car. Driving back out of the village, we passed the sign to the Hotel Splendido. 'That's one of the world's leading hotels,' I informed you in my tour-guide fashion. You immediately turned the wheel and started driving up the steep, curvy, narrow road towards it.

'What are you doing?' I exclaimed.

'Going to have a look.' You always had such a fearless attitude towards life. You pulled up outside the entrance, jumped out and went inside. You strutted out to inform me that they had one room left – and that we were staying in it. I couldn't believe it. Us, at the Splendido!

I'll be honest, though, I found the bedroom pretty uninspiring. It had unashamedly old-fashioned Italian styling, with plain white walls and furniture that had been there for decades, although at least it had a terrace overlooking the wooded hill between the hotel and the harbour. I made us a cup of Earl Grey tea, as is my habit in the afternoon. You followed it by serving us a Campari and soda from those triangular bottles in the mini-fridge, which have way more Campari than soda. I prepared myself for dinner, thankful that I'd packed my Diane von Furstenberg wrap dress and push-up, deep-plunge bra, and as I stepped out of the bathroom, you let out one of your 'wows'. Having recently started on HRT, I was blossoming out of the low neckline. You told me to stand on the terrace so you could take my photo. It was the best photo ever taken of me. It was also the start of the most magical evening of my life.

We walked through the bar out onto the beautiful terrace, dappled with evening sun. As we were led to our table by the maître d' I could sense that all the men were looking up at me – or certainly at my décolletage. It was the one and only evening of my life when that had happened, when I was the woman who caught people's eye. I felt like I was on fire.

We had a sensational dinner on that terrace looking down to the stunning harbour below. We ate a seafood pasta that blew our minds. I had veal, you had fish, with thin-cut chips (frites Splendido!) and spinach. We drank a bottle of Sicilian Nero d'Avola, which, although it's far from the best Italian wine there is, tasted to us like nectar because the evening was so blessed. The waiters couldn't have been more attentive or polite.

Afterwards, despite me thinking you'd want to hot foot it back to the bedroom, you were taken by the ambience in the bar. In a delightfully *Casablanca* way, there was a pianist in a white dinner jacket tinkling away on the piano. You ordered an espresso and an amaretto on ice (your very naff after-dinner tipple) and another glass of wine for me. We were looking round at the other guests when the pianist nonchalantly threw out a music question. 'Can anyone tell me who recorded this song?' Little did I realise that this was the evening when I would experience the phenomenon of your musical knowledge. You answered instantly. He went on, asking one music question after another. You got them all correct. He momentarily took his hands off the keys and looked across to you. He threw down the gauntlet. 'Sir, if you get this one right, you will be the guest of the week.' You got it in one. He straightened his back. 'Sir, if you get this right, you will be guest of the month.' Bingo. Utterly stunned, he thought for a moment before he said, 'Sir, if you get this next question correct, which I very much doubt you will, you will be guest of the year.' There was a hush in the bar, followed by a respectful nod and a ripple of applause, from not only him but all the other guests, as you instantly gave the correct and utterly obscure answer. From my memory it was the name of a long-gone French singer. How many other people have been guest of the year at the Hotel Splendido? How proud I was. How amazed I was. And how very chuffed you were. The guest of the year at one of the best hotels in the world! The pianist came over to ask quietly just who on earth you were.

Soon afterwards, you knocked back your drink, held out your hand and led me back to our room – you full of swagger, me almost bursting out of my dress with pride. As you shut the door you took my face in your hands to kiss me. I can only say that what followed was the night when I peaked in my womanhood and femininity.

I know that we would have to choose that as the most intoxicatingly magical night of our lives together, as every single romantic star aligned for us. And all thanks to you turning left in your car. It was all truly Splendido.

OUR HIGHLIGHTS ...

Our first kiss.

Getting your MBE from then Prince Charles at
Buckingham Palace ... followed by lunch at Elena's L'Etoile
in Charlotte Street with Sam and Beth.

Our night at the Hotel Splendido in Portofino.

Lockdown 1 – the world left us alone and we loved
five months of doing *Sounds of the 70s* together.

Doing the Silverstone F1 grid walk in 2022 – the power,
the noise, the drivers and the celebs around us ... Woo hoo!

... AND THE LOWLIGHTS

Your cancer diagnosis – the earth collapsed beneath me.

Your emergency operation in the early hours from
peritonitis – I lay awake trying not to plan your funeral
while waiting for the surgeon to call me.

Losing *Drivetime* on Radio 2 – nothing hit you as hard in
your career while we were together.

My breast cancer diagnosis – I think you took this harder
than me because you were terrified of losing me.

Losing Darcey Dog in 2022 – she was our girl,
a dog like no other.

IF I WAS A WRITER (BUT THEN AGAIN, NO)

You are thrilled that I have a book deal. 'This is your time now,' you tell me over and over. I find you reading what I've done so far on my laptop. You ask if I mind, as if it's private. I am so thrilled by your reaction. You love how I write. You love the things I say about you – things that I should have said to your face, but I am better in written words than spoken ones. You say you'd like to write a foreword. Yes, please! Delicately, I ask if you would record it too. More than that, you say you'll interview me. Today is the day we said we would do it, but instead, you sleep all day. You ignore your lunch tray. You don't want anything except my hand, which you grip as I sit next to you on the bed. The recording has to wait. Another corner has been turned. I look at your sleeping face and wonder just how empty it will feel when you're not here, and whether we will actually make that recording.

This week we watch the new Bruce Springsteen documentary *Road Diary*. It covers the build-up to the last tour and tour itself, the one we saw in Dublin. It fills our hearts to see this, to understand why he chose the set list, to meet his band. As it ends you say, 'I do have one sadness … that I will never play Bruce Springsteen on the radio again.' It is a rare moment of self-pity. It reminds me of something Richard Allinson said when we had supper once. He said, 'If any of us DJ's put on Springsteen's "Born to Run" it sounds great. When YOU put it on, Johnnie, it sounds unbelievable. You bastard!' How can it be that a song would sound different when you play it? That one comment shows me how much you have enjoyed sharing your songs. It's been your driving force and now that has gone.

It's hardly surprising you've gone down another level. Mandie, your other favourite district nurse besides Emma, says she expected this, that you will plateau now. I wonder just how many steps down and plateaus there are going to be. I take Mandie to the sitting room to show her your cards and she sheds a tear. She's always been a fan. The one fan who gets to see you in your increasingly vulnerable state.

A few days later and you do interview me. You are sitting up in bed and I am sitting on your wheelchair next to you. You're going to do an interview based on my eight favourite songs. You have my list of songs and that's it. You don't need any notes to say your introduction or ask your questions. And in this half-hour, here is what I learn: that you have taken my life on board; you have listened; you really do know me so well, so much deeper than anyone else. I answer your questions as if we're having supper together. I'm probably a bit too cocky and bold. I know I would have been more circumspect in a studio with someone else, but I feel so safe with you. I am utterly honest. You get the answers from the true me, right down to my core. It is a wonderful final gift from you. I just hope I like my answers when I hear it.

Such is our level of relief and the resultant exhaustion since you stopped Radio 2 that I am pushing visitors away. The very LAST thing I can deal with is giving my very little remaining energy to making small talk. I want to treasure this time with you. It's the first time in our marriage that we've been truly free to be us, and I love it. The vibe at home has changed: it's gentler, more in control. You lie in bed all day and I bring you meals, coffee, your pills. I sit in your wheelchair for catch-ups and to hear what the day's fan mail reveals. Such beautiful sentiments are being sent to you, and I love that you have time to read them all. 'This one's special,' you say and quote the most heartfelt, grateful and beautiful lines. You get up just before supper so you can have it with me at the table, before we then watch an hour of TV – *Rivals*, *The Diplomat* and *MasterChef: The Professionals* are the current selection.

I relent on a guest. For weeks Emily Eavis has been texting to say she wants to bring Michael Eavis over. I push her away while we approach the final show and the week after, but she is gently persistent and suggests this Friday. I cancel my flu jab and agree. I go into guest mode. The house is immaculate; a cake is made; candles are lit. We talk about where we should sit as Michael himself isn't too agile.

What transpires is the funniest visit of them all. Michael cannot get out of the car (it took a huge man to get him in it), so I get an oxygen tank, find a cannula, wrap you up in a jacket, scarf and flat cap, and out you wheel to greet Michael. It's like a reunion of war veterans – two old codgers sharing memories. It seems you are both on your third wife. Michael tells us he's ninety and stresses that he's just a farmer at heart. I bring out mugs of tea and cake. Nick, Emily's lovely husband, grabs a garden table and we have our first outdoor tea party. We share our great moments at Glastonbury, and they all absorb these with delight – Neil Young smashing up his guitar in 2009; I say that we were at the side of the stage and the bass player's wife said, 'Neil is loving this.'

'How can you tell?' I asked.

'He always smashes his guitar when he's happy.' Emily loves this story. Apparently, the great man may return for 2025, though the contract isn't signed yet. To my relief Nick asks if he can take a photo. My phone is in my pocket; I've been hoping for such an opportunity but I'm too polite to ask. We move the table and you precision drive your wheelchair, reversing towards Michael so you're in a photo-ready position. I love it. Two hugely important figures in the British music scene, grandfathers of it almost, together for the final time. It feels like a bit of history. Michael's final words to me, just before they drive off, are, 'It's been incredible really.' I tell him it has been magical, because it has. You have to have a large sprinkling of magic to create a phenomenon like Glastonbury. As they drive away, they all wave with the enthusiasm of young children. And as we come back into the warm and incredibly tidy house, we feel that some of Michael's Glastonbury stardust has been sprinkled on us. It's been one of the best and certainly most original of visits we've had. I will always be grateful that Emily persisted.

We are in such a lovely, stress-free time. We're more secluded. Safe from external forces … Until I get a call from my brother Martin. He wants to tell me that my mother, *Mutti*, is changing her will. Briefly I wonder if she's leaving me something extra in recognition of my devoted caring for you. However, I joke, as I do, 'Is she taking me out of it?' and as it transpires – she is. She's giving it all to the grandchildren instead of her four children. It's admirable to think about the next generation. And because my siblings all have at least two children each, so their bloodlines will benefit, they are happy. Even the widowed daughters-in-law of my deceased brothers are benefitting. The only one who isn't is me.

I think I'm doing really well at the moment, but with this news I learn that it doesn't take much to floor me. You can't believe it. 'Oh, Tigs. All you do is give. How can she do that to you, and now of all times?'

Why now? The first month when we have no income and I'm wondering how long my little savings pot will manage to keep us going. There's a perception in the family that we're loaded, so I imagine she thinks I don't need any help, but it's not the money – even though it would be helpful – it's the massive symbolism. There is no doubt that within families we slip back into the same roles that we've had since childhood. I suddenly feel like a very hurt youngest child. I cannot sleep when I go to bed as I'm crying too much. I cry on waking.

When I finally pick myself up after two days I call her. 'Hello, darling' – breezy as ever. In my mother's life there is no conflict, no raised voices. Everything is *marvellous*. Her answer to any problem is: 'I'm praying for you Darling' which is wonderful of her, and yet …

It isn't long into our chat that I raise the thorny issue. She is shocked as she honestly doesn't think she's done anything to get upset about. 'It's not my fault I'm childless. It's hard enough, not having kids' I blub. She tells me that I am emotional. Too emotional. And then comes the revelation, the sentence that makes her behaviour towards me make sense. She tells me that when I married you, everything changed, because I was so swept up in your busy life. She was the one who brought me up to be a devoted wife, but it has been at a cost to her and me. She just doesn't understand our world or life. I'm not sure if she disapproves of us, or whether it's her dislike of music and fame, but it is a revelation. Not least because it is an admission of her subconscious distancing from me that began two decades ago.

I have gone from being at the centre of my family to the outside.

So not only have I lost my career, fertility and identity due to our marriage, but I've lost some of my family status too! It's been quite a price. Oh, Johnnie, I should be weeping but I'm not. I don't even have a G&T in my hand, although I could kill for one. I almost feel euphoric that a missing piece of a jigsaw puzzle has been put in place. I have not invented her gentle rejection of me over these years. It's real. I heard Mutti speak her truth. And I am so happy that she did. Indeed, it's incredible.

She agrees to rethink, suggests I should be treated like a grandchild, and thus I would get an eleventh rather than a quarter. Sorry to be so mercenary, but I'm making a point. (For the record, I believe my worth has ended up as equal to two grandchildren. I am happy with this. My existence has been recognised and that's all I wanted. And she'll probably outlive me anyway!)

I'm not sure how I would have coped with this scenario without your love, support and understanding. It makes me realise how alone I will be without you. You may be a bed-ridden Puffing Billy, but you're still my rock. In the words of Bruce, 'If I should fall behind, wait for me.'

I do see the irony. It wouldn't have happened had I not met you, but being with you makes it bearable, and because of it I have learned so much about being a human. I have concluded that families are there to teach us. I wonder how she would have reacted if I'd married a royal, an aristocrat or an actor like Hugh 'Lord Grantham' Bonneville. Is it because you were a motorbike-riding music DJ who once went to rehab that she cannot understand our lives? Oh, I'd love to know, because honestly, she always refers to you as 'Dear Johnnie' so I know she likes you.

Thinking about Lord Grantham, of our many recent guests, he was a particular delight. 'I'd love to come and tell Johnnie what a wonderful actor I am for an hour!' You laugh heartily and are delighted to see him. There's such a difference between seeing people publicly and at home. He's so human with you. So open. Funny. Real. We talk about love and pain. We've all been through it, put others through it. He's going to do *Uncle Vanya* on stage in San Francisco and Washington. That I would love to see. Sadly, you certainly can't. Fortunately, though, you will be able to see *Paddington in Peru*, and you can't wait. Hugh leaves me with beautiful flowers, the warmest hug and a message later: 'You two are an inspiration to the rest of us.' Crikey. Lord Grantham … I wonder what Mutti would think.

'Surely these are the last,' you say. It's almost three weeks since your final show. More than 200 cards have been moved from our overcrowded shelf into a basket – the basket of love and gratitude. Again and again I give thanks that you have the time to reap all these rewards. Your timing has been perfect, but on a day like today, when you are not well, you sleep and sleep deeply. You are lost to me, and when you are like this I wonder whether this is the start of the final decline.

This week is an experiment – a possible-avoidance-of-a-care-home experiment. Vanessa, a well-respected carer, has come to live in and look after you so I can have a week to recover. You stop your two-day-long sleep and perk up just as she arrives and just before I leave. My goodbye is breezy and jokey. I come and say it twice for good measure and then tear off to Careys Manor Hotel & SenSpa in the New Forest to wallow in a hydrotherapy pool for two days.

You text me within an hour of my departure. You miss me. We text and text. You love the contact – we both do. You wish you were sitting opposite me for supper in the Zen Garden restaurant. I order pad Thai because that's what you'd have.

I come to London for the rest of the week. I had visions of seeing so much culture, but it's cold and I'm deeply tired. This morning I don't wake till 10.30 a.m. and I spend the day on the sofa. You report snow in Dorset. Too cold to smoke a fag, you tell me. I am sure I will have lots of texts from you, but there are none so I send you several. You don't reply. You must be asleep. At 6.07 p.m. Vanessa texts me to say you have slept all day. We stay in regular contact. I get takeout black cod from OKA in Primrose Hill village because it's your favourite dish and I'm eating it for you. For the second time this week. It's gone 10 p.m. and you are still sound asleep. This is new behaviour. A resounding dread fills me … I have always felt you will go when I least expect it. On Monday, when I left you, I certainly did not expect it, and this evening it hits me truly for the first time: at some point soon you will not be there. It's too intolerable to contemplate. You are my soulmate. Yes, I hate being tied to our restrictive life and not being able to go out together, but I have not yet truly thought how it will be without you. I'm scared, Duke. Don't go. Not yet. Not when I'm away from you. Vanessa tells me to get some sleep. She says it's important. She will contact me in the morning if you're still sleeping.

Of course I am fitful. I cannot fall asleep. At 11.15 p.m. my phone buzzes. Dread. But it's you. You have just woken. The relief is … indescribable. I thought you were exiting, but you have revived.

You had guests yesterday – the first ones without me there. Vanessa points out that you perform for guests, but it leaves you depleted. It's now taking at least a day and a half for you to recover from a visit.

I return to you, despite Storm Bert trying to stop me. It takes nearly six hours from London to home as the rail network goes into meltdown. It is so wonderful to be reunited. You can relax again, because I'm here. I know you've missed me, but I am sure the break and seeing a modicum of culture and friends was what I needed. You get that. You're generous in spirit – still.

The 'cuckoo' has been with us most of this year. Next to your bed is a doorbell, and wherever I am is the receiver. We elected on the cuckoo call as the least offensive sound it creates, and it has been invaluable all year. Tonight, the cuckoo calls. I sit bolt upright in bed, a dream violently interrupted, and I am struggling through the black of my bedroom to get to you. You apologise, but also proudly say it's the first time you've had to get me up in the dead of night. We're eleven months into this caper, so you are right to be proud. I hold you, and gently suggest that having an amaretto on ice and a black coffee after two glasses of red wine is probably not a great idea any more. You agree, but watching Knock Out week of *MasterChef*, as we were, can whet the palate. I tuck you back into bed, with fresh PJs on, and lots of blankets as it's the coldest night of the year. I cannot sleep again, not after that rude awakening. I go back to check on you, and you are sleeping like a baby, despite the sound of the new, even louder and more powerful oxygen concentrator.

I am due to go to Shropshire this weekend for my (disinheriting) mother's ninety-fourth birthday. A friend from Dublin, Kara, who asked if she can visit, has bravely agreed to come and stay and look after you, but now, still in the dark of the night, I wonder if it's safe to leave you. I cannot expect anyone other than a paid carer or nurse to deal with what I have dealt with tonight. You are going downhill, and I think my place is here.

Vanessa, experienced and psychic, has a debrief with me. She calls you a fighter, says you are fiercely independent. You wouldn't let her bath you. I am happy that this most intimate part of our caring journey you save for me. She says unless you get an infection you will be with me for Christmas. She thinks you will let go after that. *Maybe* you will get to New Year. We both know you won't make your eightieth in March. It's not even mentioned. For now, I know I must treasure each day. My family accept that by your side is where I should be. Anything else creates too much anxiety for me.

I shop online these days – who doesn't? – and I'm very excited about a pink moleskin suit that has just arrived from Seasalt. I model it for you. 'WOW, WOW, WOW!' you say, clapping your hands together. 'When are you wearing that?'

'Your funeral,' I quip, and you laugh out loud. FANTASTIC! Your laughter reverberates around the room, making me laugh too. I make you laugh quite often at the moment. You are a great audience, and your laugh both on- and off-air is wonderful, genuine, infectious. That is something I will miss hugely. I know radio listeners already are. People keep telling me that Sunday afternoons just aren't the same without you.

If we had a graph of this year, my energetic and emotional line would be at an all-time low. I'm in a perfect storm of exhaustion, domestic chaos, technical issues on the post-production of the short film, concern for you and having to scrub your carpet clean after an accident (while incidentally you happily watch F1 Qualifying sat up in bed above me). I'm too tired for my exercise class. My body aches. I'm a mess. You look at me from your bed when I bring your mid-morning coffee and biscuit and say, 'I'm worried about you, Duch. You're always so full of energy. There must be something wrong with you.' I mean, there, right there, my darling, you show a complete lack of understanding of what this year is doing to me. It's not just that I have to do everything in the house and garden, and run around looking after you, clearing up after your accidents, helping you dress, bathing you and unwinding oxygen tubes that get trapped in your wheelchair wheels. It is the emotion, the stress, the being trapped and the constant sense of anxiety about you. Alone in the kitchen I cry like a little girl who feels sorry for herself.

What I realise I miss, apart from our external life together, is hugs. It's a very real consequence of being in a wheelchair. We're at different levels all day. You can't steal up on me as you used to wrap yourself around me. You'd probably floor me with the footrest and your arms wouldn't reach. It's been such a tough couple of weeks for me, my resilience to knocks is diminishing. I'm not held by anyone and I need to be. I'm not sure how much you see me now, except at night when I kiss you goodnight and you tell me how beautiful, young or lovely I look. But I tell you how hard it is that you can no longer come and hold me when I need it. You push up the wheelchair arms, fold up the footrest and open your arms to me. I lean down and we hold each other for an age. It's beautiful. But my main thought is how thin you are now.

It's the 340th bedtime of the year. That's a lot of wheeling in the commode – renamed Ethel – getting your water and pills, putting your hearing aids in their charging pod, folding down your bedding so you can easily get in, changing your clothing, tucking you in, turning down the oxygen machine once your levels are back up to at least 80 and kissing you goodnight. Tonight, I fall on the bed next to you and say I am going to sleep there. You say that would be lovely, but we both know it won't work. I need decent sleep. I'm hardly drinking now, not eating sugar, exercising more – anything to keep up my strength because I need every ounce I can muster.

You have something very exciting to share – an audio message. As a man who is so cool and nonchalant about praise or adulation, I can only assume that it's from Bruce Springsteen. You get up and wheel into the main room. I am sitting at the dining-room table writing one of our very few Christmas cards, to Mutti. 'I want your complete attention,' you tell me. You ask for the little Bluetooth speaker to make sure it's loud. I'm actually full of excited anticipation – the Boss really would be something. I hope my smile didn't drop too far as I realised it was in fact Brian Aldridge from *The Archers*. I mean, it was hilarious, because the actor who plays him, Charles Collingwood, remained in character, and you were utterly delighted by it. But there was also something about one important radio figure recognising another and that I believe is why you were so chuffed. *The Archers* was one of the things you introduced me to, incredibly.

Now *I* have something to share. My short film, *The Kitchen Garden*, starring Ramon Tikaram and Pippa Haywood, is complete. The editing, grading, titles, music composition and sound mixing are all done. The fact that

I've managed to do this while keeping our show on the road is no small miracle. You wheel yourself to our big table, and I line up the film on my laptop and press play. You cannot believe it – the beauty of it, the lead man being in a wheelchair (your manual one, which I borrowed. You were of course the inspiration for him being disabled), the honesty of the performances, the hope, the beautiful, searing music at the end. You cry. You can't believe that I wrote, produced and directed this little gem. And I am SO PROUD that finally you get to see something I have written, which has been realised. We both know that my film script for *ANTONIA* has had to be pushed to the back burner, just as it was gaining momentum, but this I squeaked out. Honestly, it means so very much to me that you see it. You will never see *ANTONIA*, which has been with us our entire marriage – me beavering away in dogged belief and hope. This is a teaser for that film and so at least, as a reward for your great patience with me and my dream, you have a sweetener to enjoy. I go to bed tonight thinking if I never direct another thing it won't matter – because I've nailed this one and you love it. It makes my heart swell with pride.

In the spring earlier this year, when they announced that the final delayed episodes of *Yellowstone* would be aired in November, I didn't dare tell you as I knew – yes, knew – that you would miss them, yet we have just finished them – together – along with the final of *Strictly Come Dancing*. Despite you saying that Christmas 2023 was your last, this year's tree is up and tomorrow, on the shortest day, we will celebrate our twenty-second wedding anniversary.

You feel you've gone down another notch. Two really bad panic attacks this week have you as worried as you have been all year. I go into overdrive and get a GP round (the first since January!), speak to our palliative nurse Angel Caroline and the district nurses. Sometimes I think all you need is some reassurance. Who wouldn't be nervous of their moment of demise? Both the doc and Caroline say that you aren't going anywhere yet. Indeed, Caroline and I have a heart to heart. With the greatest compassion, she hopes for your sake that you will suddenly get pneumonia, as then it would be over in days. The alternative is a long, drawn-out decline – as you are already in – going on for months. Dignity will reduce; living will get even harder. You've started saying that you would happily take a pill to end it all. Not before Christmas, obviously, but you say this week you think the end of January will be your time. The not knowing, for both of us, is the biggest challenge there is. If you do get an infection, you will be gone within days and I will be left in shock. Released from caring yes, but facing the unimaginable, which is you not being here.

OUR TOP TWENTY DRAMA SERIES

Breaking Bad
The Bureau
My Brilliant Friend
Chernobyl
Mad Men
Borgen
1883
Yellowstone
The English
The Crown
War and Peace
The Marvellous Mrs Maisel (first two series)
Deutschland 83/86/89
Shōgun
Daisy Jones & the Six
The Bridge
The Queen's Gambit
The White Lotus
Succession
The Morning Show

MY DUKE (OF EARL)

I have so often wondered why we made a good couple. Indeed, have we made a good couple? People tell us so. We've always been told about our obvious deep love for each other – apparently, it touches and inspires others. Us! Sometimes I think we've conned them all, for I swear we've had as many rows as everyone else.

When I stand back and look at you as objectively as I can, I am amazed by you. You have been such a contradiction: a mixture of huge strengths and weaknesses. But of this I am very proud – the difference in you between our meeting and now is immense. I'd like to think I've helped you to feel better about yourself. A lot better. 'Loving You Makes Me a Better Man' – you have always quoted that song; maybe that's the love that people see.

That September in 2001 when we met, you were financially challenged. Indeed, you were over £40,000 in debt, as you'd spent huge amounts settling your legal bills after your *News of the World* sting. You didn't own anything other than an old second-hand Saab and a Harley-Davidson Fatboy.

You lived in a shitty rented flat. You were still in a period of questioning, having not long left rehab. You were totally clean – no booze, no fags and certainly no cocaine. You were on a spiritual quest; somewhat serious, introverted, quite insecure, with a hugely developed sense of guilt. There was no doubt that you'd been attracted to the sort of women who made you feel bad about yourself, and made you feel guilty. You used to talk with Gordon about the 'Madonna and Whore' syndrome. Using your imagery, you had been excited by 'whores', but your soul said you needed a 'Madonna' to survive. In I walked. No wonder it was a clash of directions for you at the start of our relationship. It was part of your journey. You didn't know what you wanted, which is why I was always understanding about the first cancelled wedding. You were not ready. I don't believe we would have survived if we'd tied the knot then. The Temple of Doom would have been apt. The five-month wait between July and December 2002 was crucial to us succeeding, for in that time you learned more about me, and let yourself go and fall in love with this 'straight' – who wasn't straight at all!

It felt to me as if no one had ever told you 'how wonderful you are', to steal Gordon's lyric. You had been hearing for too long what was bad about you and not what was good. The truth is that you had so much good in you, but you had to see it. I even thought you were paranoid when you said you were convinced your phone was being tapped (and as it happens, it was, but we decided not to act). You seemed at sea. Your shitty rented flat pretty much summed up what you felt you deserved.

I've watched you grow in confidence, relax, embrace the good in life and trust others. In turn, I have become more worldly wise and very much stronger. Possibly trust is the key to love. You could trust me. Whatever you threw at me, you knew that while I might justifiably explode in rage and get upset, I would calm down once I had caught my breath, because we had some unspoken, soul-level connection. I was, and always would be, your greatest supporter and ally. Something in you knew that down to your core.

So often the upset was about smoking, which I fought tooth and nail for you to avoid. I learned that you were probably smoking all the time we've been together, but far behind my back. I thought I was married to a non-smoker. I have thrown my wedding ring at you and left home over fags, and I have to ask myself just why I was so incensed by them. You have been so sick throughout our marriage, and so many people, including me, have sacrificed so much to keep you going. I read smoking as the hugest insult to us all. What a dragon I have been, but really, I was just the person who wanted her soulmate to last as long as possible.

You've always been a profligate spender – money literally burned a hole in your pocket. You have bought masses and masses of completely unnecessary things. If there was money in your account or wallet, you had a deep compulsion to get rid of it – the total opposite of careful me. I tried so many arguments with you – like saving the planet, or thinking about me when you've gone. It didn't touch you. Your attitude was, 'There'll always be a way to survive,' as if survival was the only goal. It does mean, however, that you were hugely generous to many. From *Big Issue* sellers and waiters, through to the charity coffers at Salisbury District Hospital and Carers UK. I've secretly loved that generosity of spirit you've had. I believe it shows your very great goodness of heart. Your financial philosophy (if that isn't too grand a concept for a spending addict) seems to be akin to the one Jesus would hold – not your words, but my take on you. I'm sure this attitude has been a lesson you were here to teach me: not to be worried, to let it flow, to let life carry you. Because it will. As Jean the medium once said to me, there is no money in heaven. It's very much an earthly concern. No wonder you loved all-inclusive resorts. They were heaven on earth for you!

It has been complex, being married to someone who could get so lost in his own shell. A true radio man. Someone who could either be fantastic fun socially or utterly silent. It was always a challenge going out to supper parties. How would you be that evening? Which Johnnie would they see? The ebullient friendly one, or the one who sloped off to the nearest sofa and slept? It was usually the latter, so I had to work hard at supper parties, making excuses or trying to fill the entertainment gap. Close friends accepted and knew this; others could be offended, and we would not be invited back. Oh and when the dreaded question came from a person around the table, 'So Johnnie, how did you get into radio?' AAAAGH! I must confess we would both want to fall head first into our plate of food. Inwardly I'd be screaming, 'Bloody Wiki him!' Honestly, when you started working weekends only, it was fabulous to have the excuse that 'Johnnie needs an early night'.

Your capriciousness certainly kept me on my toes, but equally you'd take a certain amount of shit from me. 'You cannot do that, Johnnie!' or 'Do NOT say that on-air!' (especially if invited onto Radio 4). And you would listen – almost. You seemed to think I was wise.

Your amazing talents on radio gave you a confidence in the studio alone. I sometimes think the best radio people are those with deep questions and insecurities, Kenny Everett being the most brilliant example. Would you have been so good on-air if you were cocksure in the rest of your life?

I saw your strength when you gave me advice. You had the ability to stand back from my situations and give such strong guidance, because you have always been intrinsically stronger than me in spirit. You have survived so many bombs going off in your life; you have been an instinctive fighter, never giving up. You may have surrounded yourself with your petty addictions like smoking, shopping and conspiracy theories, but you would drop all that rubbish when I'd say, 'Duke – I need your help. What should I do?' You could read a situation as well as anyone, and you pushed me to be stronger.

Why do I love you? Apart from knowing your soul … it's because, just as you needed some 'straightness' in your life from me (which I would call 'grounding', because as I keep telling you, I'm really not that straight compared with most), I needed some wildness from you. I love your spirit, your laughter, your courage, your naughtiness, your ability to lead me astray as if it was good for me, your morality, your deep kindness and above all your humility, despite the incredibly successful man you have been. Fame has never gone to your head. Your feet have remained on the ground, and you treat everyone as equals. These are great traits, and you are a fine – if complicated and occasionally flawed – example of a human being. You have taught me so much. You have been the greatest teacher in my life. And that's quite apart from your taste in music. How could I not love you?

CALLING TIME

Something is going on. Is it the winter solstice? Two years ago you fell out of a helicopter at this time. Last night, in your increasingly independent fashion, you went to turn on your bedroom oxygen machine instead of asking me to do it. The result was that you totally dislodged your bed, pulled the bedding off it and collided with your wingback chair, getting tied up in the tubes from not just one, but two machines. You actually pulled two sections of tubing apart. I was charging round after you, trying to untie your tubes from the wheelchair and put them back together. It was an impossible task. For five minutes our world was in chaos and you had no oxygen. I was furious at you for putting me into that state of panic and yourself in danger, just because you want to be independent.

Tonight, as I put the final touches on our twenty-second-anniversary dinner, I hear an almighty crash. I run out of the kitchen to find you prostrate across the hall corridor. I throw myself on the floor next to you in my leopard-skin trousers and sexy black top, with tousled hair, bright red lips – and an apron. You're wearing just a T-shirt and pants. I cannot understand how you got to be there, and neither can you. You are metres away from your wheelchair or bed. As the salmon en croute burns in the oven, I am trying to assess you, and then get you up. You have spoken, and you don't appear to have broken anything, but your elbow is cut in two places and there is blood all over the blanket I rest your head on. After fifteen minutes of trying to elevate you, I have to call on my neighbours. Clare comes round and together, very slowly, we get you back up onto the wheel-chair. You mutter something about wanting to look nice for our dinner. You've given yourself a hell of a shock – plus a bump on the head. After dinner, when you can't face the gorgeous Chablis, we watch the final episode of *The Day of the Jackal*. You ask if there are two men on the hillside. There is just one. I fret. Do you need the paramedics to check you over? You say you don't. You, like me, are afraid of you being carted off, as you may never return.

We get you to bed; it's slow. 'God bless,' we say to each other. 'Happy anniversary.' And as I come to bed I wonder if your prediction last December that that would be your final Christmas may still prove to be true.

You sleep deeply for over twelve hours. I'm concerned so I call the paramedics, but they won't take you in as you don't want to ever go to hospital again. They are slightly concerned by your double vision last night, your long sleep and your general fogginess. They are great and give me guidance: I need to get a treatment escalation plan sorted with the doctors. The issue of you falling is a new concern, previously unthought of. It's always been an infection that was a threat. You could get a brain bleed if you hit your head again. Clearly, your reducing mobility is now an issue. The lead paramedic speaks to me in the kitchen and gently implies that I should be ready for anything to happen. She also tells me I'm doing a great job of looking after you. It means a lot to me. And after they go, you sleep again.

When you wake at 6.30 p.m. you have no idea if it's day or night, or what day of the week it is. You ask where everyone is – have they all gone to bed? I explain that it's just us who live here and you seem relieved. You ask questions about *The Day of the Jackal*'s final episode. You don't remember a single scene. You ask what I had for supper and I explain it is yet to be cooked, so you come and join me for it. You're a liability in your wheelchair. You crash into furniture, you almost push the kitchen island over and you start loading logs into the lit woodburning stove. I get panicky. You could blow us all up with your oxygen on. I actually start to get worried. You don't speak, you just drive that bloody wheelchair around, creating havoc. You go outside for a fag – you refuse your jacket, although I manage to put your cap and scarf on you. As you sit outside on a cold, wet night in your PJs and a thick cardigan, I have a strong sense that you're having your final smoke. By the time I get you to bed I slump on your bedroom wingback chair with my head in my hands. I can't cope alone anymore. I say out loud, 'I need help now.' I leave your door and mine open, and spend the night fitfully tossing around and listening to your breathing. I go in to check on you four times. I feel you're as close to the end as you have ever been. By 5 a.m. I am too exhausted to keep up the vigilance. I shut the doors and manage three hours of sleep.

When one of the district nurses comes in to check on you in the morning she asks if I need some home care help. It's the first time I've been offered this, and as we have totally dropped the idea of putting you in a home because you are so frail, I answer, 'YES, I absolutely do.' I've carried this on my own for 357 days (a year, minus eight days) so, yes, I need back-up. By the afternoon I am told that as from tomorrow I will have someone coming in for forty-five minutes a day for the next fortnight. I've no idea how it will work out and what the carer will do, but at least it means I can go and get the turkey, as right now I dare not leave you at all. Eating has been hard because your side hurts so much, so now you have your first NHS liquid meal. I don't know if this is a big gear change, or whether you just need to recover from the fall. I realise that I've picked up a chesty cough. I need sleep more than anything.

Despite your declaration that last Christmas would be your final one, we manage a lovely Christmas Day 2024, with my brother Martin and his wife, Kate, coming to cook us a delicious lunch. The stars that they are, and have been all year. You keep going until 6 p.m. and then feel really ill.

Boxing Day, my birthday, is one of my happiest. At supper we are once again the gang of six: d'Arcy, Gary, Jane and Charles arrive with lasagne, cake, profiteroles and a lot of indecently good champagne and wine. Along with cold turkey, baked spuds and salad, we have a right old feast. Even though you start the evening on the edge of proceedings and in tears because you forgot to order a cake (Jane rescued that), you slowly join in and we all have fantastic political banter round the table. Right versus Left: Sir Keir and 'Rachel from Accounts/Complaints' getting plenty of stick from you and Charles; Gary standing up for the environment; d'Arcy saying give Labour time, and me just loving having my besties around our table on my birthday. I couldn't be happier. Jane lights the candles on the cake, while you hold the plate with such pride. Do you believe the candles are burning for you? Or is it your relief that I had a birthday cake after all? I kiss your forehead. Jane, being the talented documentary film director that she is, snaps a photo. It turns out to be your final photo. You look so pleased with yourself.

On Saturday, 28 December I arrange to go to Jane's for a birthday tea with friends so you can have some time alone with one of your relatives. It's all been carefully orchestrated. Just before I leave you tell me the guest is not coming, so on what turns out to be the last day of your life up and about, you sit alone. I cannot cancel as the tea has been arranged for me, and when I return you look forlorn. 'Duke!' I throw my arms around you. You tell me you feel tired and want to go to bed. In the future it breaks my heart that you spent your final afternoon of normality all alone.

So many lasts have happened, and yet at the time we are oblivious to the fact that they would be later labelled with that adjective. Our last intimacy, our last proper hug, our last laugh together, our last supper together at the table, your last afternoon in our sitting room … If we had known they were 'lasts', would we have treasured these precious moments more?

A year ago today we were having an abstemious day as we were preparing to leave early in the morning for your live *Sounds of the 70s* show at Wogan House – your last at that studio, and your last ever live show. This evening I sit on the beautiful wingback chair at the end of your bed and watch you propped up on pillows, trying to eat a crustless egg and cress sandwich, as that has always been one of your go-to sick meals. You haven't eaten or drunk for the past two days and have been so worryingly sick that there have been two doctors and a district nurse (lovely Emma) here, and Cindy, the new carer, has been up five times today. Out of the goodness of her heart. Last night as I bathed you, you said you'd like to go to the local cottage hospital in Shaftesbury for rehydration and some care. Today we learn you are too acutely ill to go there, it being such a small hospital. They will only take you when you are end-of-life, and Emma judges you not to be at that stage. Yet. Though you could easily slip there. It's Salisbury District Hospital or home, and we both know the answer to that. The home care has been increased to twice a day from tomorrow because you are declining. Gorgeous, kind women, Debbie and Cindy, will wash you and change your sheets. It is such a help to me to have them come in that I tell Debbie she is the greatest Christmas present ever.

This evening, as you drop in and out of sleep, having managed just two tiny fingers of egg sandwich, I wonder how much longer you will fight. I ask if I should contact your kids. You flatly reply, 'No.' Shouldn't we ask Beth to come over? 'No.' Either you don't feel as ill as you look and seem, or you're just too weak for visitors. I have realised this about you – if I had to say you were a radio man or a family man, I would definitely say the former.

Tomorrow a hospital bed will arrive for a second time. This time it will have to stay because of the carers. And there is talk of a catheter to make life easier. These are markers – markers that you are slowing down considerably, whether it be in the next two days or the next six weeks. You are so much weaker than you were before the fall eight days ago, and I assume that strength will not return. As I kiss you goodnight we share a little loving joke. I think about saying, 'Enjoy your final night in this bed,' but for once I hold back. You don't need that reminder.

I hear you cry out. It's still dark, being only 6.40 a.m., so I bash into furniture as I run to your room, forgetting we have lights in my panic. You are in distress, half out of bed, your bedding half off it. You have pulled out your oxygen tube. I stick the cannula back up your nostrils and turn you up to MAX. You don't make any sense. You're trying to communicate with your hands while I try to get the oximeter on your finger. I can't get a reading. I give you a shot of Oramorph to calm you. I lie on the bed behind you and hold you, stroking your hair. I know instinctively that this is it, but your determination to survive is deep. You want me to call an ambulance, and honestly, this one time, I wish I'd ignored you, as I wish I had stayed right there in that loving embrace. However, I do run to get the phone, and I hold your hand as I speak to the 999 woman. My two-minute-long conversation goes from, 'I think my husband is dying …' to, 'I think my husband has died.' She asks me to remove the pillows, straighten your body and tilt back your head, but I know it's too late. You're not breathing. She asks me to watch your chest and tell her each time it rises. I am silent. She says she's sorry for my loss. Your death is recorded at 6.50 a.m. In the end my final words to you were not, 'I'm bloody knackered'. Neither were they, 'I love you' or 'thank you' or 'goodbye my love'. They were me asking incredulously, 'You want me to call an ambulance?!'.

I thought you were invincible. You have the spirit of someone who would never die, and yet here you are before me, silent. Still. Gone. Elsewhere. My only consolation is that I was with you, though I honestly cannot say exactly when you slipped away.

It's New Year's Eve. One year exactly since your last live show. Day 365 of being so intensely ill. Bless you, my darling Duke. You are released, my love. I can't quite believe it. How will my life be without you?

THE TEN MAIN THINGS
I MISS ABOUT YOU

Your infectious laughter.

The warmth of your body holding me.

Watching you broadcasting live in the studio.

Our evenings together – supper and a streamer.

You driving me (your chauffeur name was 'Baines').

Going on holiday together.

Your belief in me.

Complaining about *The Archers!*

The exciting invites.

Your voice on the radio (and in that I am not alone).

WHAT I THINK ARE YOUR MOST IMPORTANT TRACKS

(Guessed by me posthumously)

The Shirelles
WILL YOU STILL LOVE ME TOMORROW
One of your favourites. You would melt when you heard it.

Percy Sledge
WARM AND TENDER LOVE
Your last track on your Radio Caroline shows.

Sam & Dave
SOUL MAN
You loved them and their energy, and particularly this song.

Beatles
ALL YOU NEED IS LOVE
The first song you played when you became a 'criminal' continuing to broadcast on Radio Caroline after the Marine, &c., Broadcasting (Offences) Act became law on 14 August 1967.

Lou Reed
WALK ON THE WILD SIDE
*Your most risqué Record of the Week at Radio 1, which saved
Lou Reed's career. Decades later, when he learned that you were the
'DJ in Europe' who had championed it, he said that you had paid
his rent over all these years.*

Bruce Springsteen
THE RIVER
*I struggle to choose the right track, but you loved his music above
everyone else's. Indeed, I think you recognised his soul, both of you
searching yet sometimes struggling to grasp happiness, and
finding solace from that struggle in music.*

Todd Snider
ALRIGHT GUY
*What you played when you came back from 'gardening leave'
after the News of the World drugs sting in 1999, pre-me.*

Jackson Browne
BEFORE THE DELUGE
*You love the soul and songwriting of JB.
I think this was your favourite.*

Elton John and Kiki Dee
DON'T GO BREAKING MY HEART
*Your last Record of the Week on Radio 1,
which led to Elton's first Number One single. You received a gold
disc, which hung on your den wall.*

Bonnie Raitt
ANGEL FROM MONTGOMERY
*You had a thing about Bonnie – the ultimate rock chick.
The 'Oh, Johnnie' jingle you used was Bonnie after you told her
on-air that you would have married her – or words to that effect.
You were too late!*

NOW

GOODBYE, MY LOVE

Without doubt, your funeral was a triumph. I know we'd discussed a few key things, like the setting for the service and wake – St Peter's Church and the Grosvenor Arms in Shaftesbury – and we'd discussed a few tracks, and who you did not want invited, but mostly you wanted to leave it to me – as you tended to do. And I'm glad you did that, as it became quite an organic production. One thing led to another as it all fell neatly and gloriously into place with ease.

The local Palida Choir who you wanted were brilliant. Yes, live music was the way to go. It's thanks to them that you came in to Joni Mitchell's 'Both Sides Now' – it was already in their repertoire. I think it was a great choice, don't you? And their version of Rani Arbo and Daisy Mayhem's 'Crossing the Bar' – you'd already heard that, and it was completely bang on for a man who started his career on a pirate radio ship. Our spiritual friend Pippa Haywood felt she saw you sat on your coffin, swinging your legs and watching them sing that. Oh, I bet you loved the laughter.

There was a lot. And weren't you touched that your old friend Rick Wakeman played his own funeral composition for you? That was the moment that got everyone, when they truly thought about you.

Getting the guest list right was a challenge. The church has so few seats, and everyone I asked came. Can you believe how many of your radio colleagues turned up? Jeremy Vine, Ken Bruce, Bob Harris, Jo Whiley, Shaun Keaveny, Simon Mayo, Tony Blackburn, Paul Gambaccini, Richard Allinson, Sally Boazman, Helen Thomas and Mark Goodier. Well, Mark had to, as he was doing half your eulogy. I hope you think we did you proud. Robert Plant and his wonderful head of hair certainly turned a few heads in Shaftesbury. As did Michael Eavis with Emily.

One of the people I'd asked to contribute was Paul Venables. He said something that has stayed with me since: 'Twenty-two years ago I was asked to read at Johnnie and Tiggy's wedding. The piece they asked me to read on that day was from a poem called 'The Invitation'. I was looking back over that reading the other day and was really struck by a particular line. It said:

It doesn't interest me who you know – I want to know if you will stand in the centre of the fire with me and not shrink back.

Well Johnnie and Tiggy, you both stood in that fire, with courage and dignity and with love. We all know that Tiggy.' I had never made that connection from our wedding day. But Paul was right. We did stand in the fire, and we never shrunk back.

I wanted more than anything to give you a good send-off, and it went ten times better than I could have imagined. It was the last thing I could do for you. It had to be good, and it was a triumph. The music was amazing, the readings fantastic, but the thing I know you will have loved the most was the seven Harley-Davidsons that waited to follow your hearse out of Shaftesbury with, as you requested, 'Born to Run' blasting out. You had no idea about the bikes. Those were thanks to our ever-loyal Sarah, our right-hand woman for so many years, who made the suggestion and arranged it.

Your funeral was full of love for you, Duke. It was a true reflection of the man you were. It was moving, funny, a bit spiritual, dignified and completely and utterly unforgettable.

P.S. Can I just say I appreciated your little stint at the end of the day. While plenty of people sensed you in church, I was too much in producer mode. But coming to bed later that night and smelling cigarette smoke in my room – bloody hell, you little bugger. Of all the ways to reveal yourself. And yes, I laughed.

TIGGY'S EULOGY

It's a brave man who asks his wife to do his eulogy. It's even braver when that man is Johnnie Walker. But Johnnie was brave. Very brave.

Twenty-two years of marriage to him was a veritable roller-coaster and, honestly, I'm still shaking from the ride. But I will say, I was never bored for one moment – even though occasionally that would have been a relief.

But Johnnie knew, no matter what challenges he put me through, I would always be his most loyal defender and protector, fighting to the hilt for him, be it with the BBC, HMRC or anyone who crossed him.

A lot has been said in the media about him being rebellious, tricky, a maverick, a rule-breaker. But today I want to focus on the brilliant things about Johnnie. And there were a lot.

Of course, we all know he was a superlative broadcaster with fantastic music taste – and his great friend Mark Goodier is going to talk about his career, so I will focus on the less-discussed sides of the man.

Let's start with his name. He was born Peter Dingley in Solihull, the fourth of five children in a family he described as neurotic. He couldn't wait to get away. And out to sea he went, where Radio England gave him a choice of jingle packages: Johnnie Walker or Boom Boom Branigan. The man had taste. But the name Peter never left him. To his family here today he is still Peter or Uncle Peter. UP for short. And it's one of the main reasons he wanted his funeral here at St Peter's – a church he always loved.

His great humour was a joy to all. He had a laugh that reverberated out as if he kept remembering how funny the joke was. On-air it was Sally Traffic who made him laugh. Off-air it was me. Even during his last depleted year, we shared much hilarity together. When a couple of months ago this suit I'm wearing arrived, I styled it for him, as I did all new clothes. 'Wow, wow, wow. That's fantastic. What have you bought it for?' 'Your funeral,' I replied, and he couldn't stop laughing. So naturally I had to wear it today. Our final joke was in the week before he died. There was talk of catheters. When I referred to his Urethra Franklin he was off, almost crying with laughter.

Johnnie was by far the best driver I know. He was fast, confident, dominant and yet safe and remarkably polite. He actually trained at Jim Russell's motor racing school and if he hadn't become a DJ, then he would have aimed for Monaco. His love of F1 continued through his life, and one of his more recent highlights was doing the grid walk at Silverstone in 2022, just before the race started. Johnnie loved energy and power, and you never feel that more than when you're stood among twenty-two F1 cars that are getting ready to race. He had few regrets in his final year, but one of them was that he wouldn't get to see Lewis Hamilton drive a Ferrari.

Johnnie had a naturally generous heart. He wouldn't just give away his last Rolo; he'd go into debt to give you an entire packet. If he saw a *Big Issue* seller he'd call them over, give them £20 and tell them he didn't need the mag because he'd already read it. He donated to many charities – the RNLI, Compassion in World Farming, the Stars Appeal at Salisbury District Hospital and, most notably, Carers UK, the charity supporting unpaid carers, of which we were proud to be co-patrons. Caring for each other through illness proved to be a dominant theme of our time together. He wasn't just generous with his money, but with his time and influence. From walking a wild section of the Great Wall of China with a group of friends, which raised over £65,000, to poetry readings, fundraising events, carers' awards, meeting other unpaid carers at events around the nation, attending tea at Parliament and getting the support of Jeremy Vine and Radio 2 during Carers Week. Johnnie was truly proud of what we achieved together, always happier talking about others in need rather than himself.

Johnnie's strength generally was something quite extraordinary. I've never known a stronger person in will, determination or belief. He almost died in the first year of our marriage during his cancer treatment. He went from a life-support machine back to the Radio 2 *Drivetime* show in four months. Time and again he had health issues – a heart attack, triple heart bypass and double pneumonia to name a few. Again and again, he would return to the studio as soon as he could. His resilience to the pitfalls and challenges of life was remarkable. He lived on 'Planet IS' and not 'Planet SHOULD', never feeling sorry for himself, just driven to keep going. This last year it was truly amazing how long he kept broadcasting. He took it to his very edge, carrying on when most would have stopped, pulling himself out of bed and putting on his performance voice before returning back to bed. It was a shock for me when he died because I didn't think he ever would. He was stoic, brave, never self-pitying. He had wonderful warrior strengths – and probably the strengths you need to be so successful in the public arena.

Despite his success, humility was a key trait of his. I think it's why he was so loved. The first time he shoved me in front of a mic, he was depping on the *Breakfast Show* for Terry Wogan. He would hand me a bunch of text messages to read out. If there was anything complimentary about him, me or the show, he crossed it out. He didn't need the flattery. Indeed, he had no concept of how popular he was. When Steve Wright died last February it was big news. Johnnie almost apologetically warned me that when he went there would hardly be any attention at all. How very wrong he was.

Timing is an art and one he had in spades. He was old school, knowing how to get up to the news without cutting off the track, working out timings fifteen minutes before the top of the hour. But his timing in life was uncannily good too. The night we met we talked about the world being spiritually bereft and how a wake-up call was needed. The next day was 9/11. We got married on the winter solstice – a symbolic day AND the longest night. We also married less than a month before his health started to decline, which on his part was superb timing. His final live show was on New Year's Eve 2023, and his death came exactly one year later, just two months after his final pre-recorded show. When Mandie the nurse came to verify his death that morning she said: 'What timing, Johnnie. New Year's Eve. That's so rock 'n' roll.' Not only was it rock 'n' roll, but Bob Harris was live that afternoon with *Sounds of the 70s* and within ten hours of his death, he had a tribute show unfolding on Radio 2. He died the day the dreaded hospital bed was arriving – so he avoided that, and his Urethra Franklin being 'catheterised'. He was also, selflessly, desperate to release me from the heavy burden of caring, and something in him must have thought Tiggy needs to start 2025 afresh. And I am grateful for that.

Spiritual wisdom was possibly his most profound strength. He had a special moment when he was in rehab on Antigua when he believed God spoke to him. While he wasn't a traditional Anglican man, his belief in God, Jesus and the afterlife was absolute. He believed that on this earth we are spirits on a human journey, here to constantly learn and improve our souls before we pass. He believed we have a preview of our life before we choose it. So whenever he upset me, he'd say, 'But, Tigs, you chose this life.' It was handy.

Well, Johnnie, if I really did choose to be with you, then I obviously wanted to learn a great deal. Through good and bad, you have significantly altered and strengthened the sweet, innocent girl you married twenty-two years ago. You have been the greatest teacher in my life. I just ask that you keep sending me your strength as I continue my journey without you.

As for you, I hope you are now reflecting on the extraordinary life you've lived. You touched so many hearts. And I will always be incredibly proud of you. God bless you, darling Johnnie. And thank you.

MARK GOODIER'S EULOGY

On the evening of 13 August 1967, aboard a beat-up former fishing boat off the Essex coast, Johnnie was broadcasting to an estimated 22 million listeners across the UK and Europe.

In Johnnie's words, 'I was frightened to death. I was exhilarated, excited. It was just incredible. I knew the moment the second hand swept past the 12 that if I said a word I'd be a criminal, liable for prosecution for the next two years, living in exile in Holland. It was a huge moment.'

Midnight arrived. Johnnie played 'We Shall Overcome', followed by a message to Harold Wilson and then the Beatles' 'All You Need Is Love'. Afterwards, they 'opened the champagne'.

This was Johnnie Walker: a maverick, of immense integrity, a man for whom it was all about the music.

This spirit would see Johnnie continue broadcasting on Radio Caroline long after it was outlawed by Harold Wilson's government, drawing crowds of 'Frinton Flashers' along stretches of the south-east coastline, beaming their headlights out into the dark waters while Johnnie played the likes of the Beatles, Otis Redding and Wilson Pickett and broadcast coded appeals to Dee Dee in London for tea. Within two days an envelope full of spliffs would arrive from Dee Dee, followed by sackfuls of PG Tips and Typhoo from the thousands of listeners. Johnnie said: 'I've never seen so many tea bags in my life.' Johnnie was doing one of the things that made him a special broadcaster – talking with, not at, the listener and building his relationship with them.

Johnnie returned to dry land in 1968 and started his longstanding relationship with the BBC with a job at Radio 1 in April '69 – a two-hour show on a Saturday afternoon. Johnnie's rebellious instincts made that relationship at times pretty colourful.

In 1976, frustrated with BBC management's insistence on playing the playlist, and only the playlist, Johnnie suggested listeners who didn't agree with his views on the Bay City Rollers could – I quote – 'take a running jump', and, having been told he was too 'into the music', quit Radio 1 and set sail for the Sunshine State.

But it wasn't plain sailing in the USA – denied a Green Card, Johnnie worked at KSAN in San Francisco for literally the love of radio, spending hours every week crafting documentaries – for no payment whatsoever – and DJing between the bands at concerts and being a promoter on the emerging Punk scene, until it was shut down by the cops.

Johnnie would return to the UK in the early Eighties – to Radio West and to Wiltshire Radio, where he honed speech radio skills that would set him up perfectly for future roles back at the BBC, at Greater London Radio, as a founding presenter on Radio 5, and Radio 1, where he'd present *The Stereo Sequence*.

Saturday afternoons were also where Johnnie landed his own show at what became his forever home, Radio 2. Johnnie was the perfect fit for a radio station that was reinventing itself – and Johnnie stayed for twenty-seven years.

After hosting *Drivetime*, and a late-Sunday-afternoon show, in 2009 Johnnie began hosting *Sounds of the 70s*, the show that would bookend his career and soundtrack many of our lives. It was the perfect show for Johnnie, one he could have done on the hoof, but one he approached with a focus, integrity, tenacity and passion right until the last.

On 27 October 2024 Johnnie presented his final *Sounds of the 70s* from his home in Dorset – my colleagues and I had produced his Sunday shows for eighteen years. We all knew how seriously unwell he was and marvelled at his spirit and strength to keep going for as long as he did.

Johnnie always knew the right songs for the occasion – that last *Sounds of the 70s* was a perfect personal selection.

On that show **Rod Stewart** spoke for many about Johnnie's contribution to radio and music:

'I have to thank you from the bottom of my heart for playing not only my songs, but the Faces and just about every rock band in the world over the years. By doing so you propelled a bunch of unknown layabouts to the top of the charts. Without your support we never may have got there.'

For today, I invited others to express how they feel:

Roger Taylor: 'Johnnie Walker was a true rarity – a powerful radio presence who truly loved the music he presented. He always seemed personally invested in it. As musicians we understood his genuine appreciation, which was rare in our business.'

Ronnie Wood: 'Whenever we sat down for an interview it was more like a chat with a dear old friend, it was never a hassle, never boring and always good fun.'

Mark Knopfler: 'The music always came first with Johnnie. There wasn't a trace of pretension about him: There was passion, humour and a deep love for people and for music, which is why he is missed by so many.'

Joan Armatrading: 'With Johnnie, it was never like doing an interview. He was so warm it was like talking with a friend about music.'

Robert Plant: 'So long, Johnnie Walker, all across the years a defender and gatekeeper of great musical taste … a cool, kind man who kept the bar high for all of us who loved him … Time roars and mocks us all … he gifted a quiet calm, groove and taste that got so many of us through.'

THE MUSIC AT YOUR FUNERAL

Joni Mitchell
BOTH SIDES NOW
Sung by the Palida Choir as your coffin was brought in.

Hymn
DEAR LORD AND FATHER OF MANKIND
... forgive our foolish ways.

GONE BUT NOT FORGOTTEN
Written and played on grand piano by Rick Wakeman.

Rani Arbo and Daisy Mayhem
CROSSING THE BAR
Sung by the Palida Choir.

Hymn
FIGHT THE GOOD FIGHT
Because you always did.

Judy Collins
AMAZING GRACE

Sung by the Palida Choir as your coffin was carried out.

Bruce Springsteen
BORN TO RUN

Blasting out from the hearse as you were driven away.

EPILOGUE

Grief is such an individual journey. I was an empty husk when we waved goodbye to Johnnie on Shaftesbury High Street back in January. I didn't have the strength for grieving then. I was not only tired, but also still in shock, I guess. I almost thought he'd never actually die, because his ability to hold on was so immense. Then, all of a sudden, he just wasn't there. All that intense caring ended in an instant. And while I had a whole year to prepare for that moment, it wasn't at all as I had imagined, and there were still things I'd forgotten to check – and I don't just mean how to turn on the TV. We had a little book that I'd asked him to put all his passcodes in, and most of these were illegible or just plain wrong! Why hadn't I gone over these with him?

At the funeral I was still dealing with the lack of rest, as well as handling the practicalities of life – like the phone call from GT, our accountant, three days after he died: 'Darling, there's no easy time to tell you this, but JW owes £42,000 in tax.' Johnnie had been forced to become PAYE by the BBC for the final twenty months of his career, and we had both assumed the tax deducted was the correct amount. It was not. To say this was a body blow is an understatement. I became like a sleuth trying to access his bank and premium-bond accounts, but they were all empty. Oh, Johnnie! There's only one thing you can do in situations like that, and that's laugh. When I met him he was over £40,000 in debt, and he left me in the same way. That's the circle of life, I guess. The small pot I had saved for us to survive on was all sent to HMRC. I genuinely believe this was one of Johnnie's lessons to me: don't worry about money. You'll always find a way to survive. Survival is currently based on selling his record collection, clothes and innumerable gadgets – thank you to my new friends on Vinted! In a way I feel more financially secure now. I know exactly what I have, and there's no risk of him buying yet more stuff he didn't need. A pair of night-driving glasses arrived exactly one week after he died. He hadn't driven for a year. I actually shouted up to the skies, 'Dear God, please tell me he hasn't got an Amazon account up there.'

I needed sleep and rest, which I got in Jamaica at an adult-only hotel called Couples that we used to go to together on Negril Beach, only now I was set the challenge of being the ONLY single person at a hotel full of romantic duos, facing head on all the fun Johnnie and I had together there in the past. While I admit to sitting at dinner with tears tumbling down my face on occasion, I couldn't have been more warmly embraced by the gorgeous staff. 'Honey

– you look beautiful on the outside this evening. How are you on the inside, baby?'

I honestly felt Johnnie close to me when I arrived. I asked him for a sign – which I quickly got. Our last trip to the Caribbean had been to Grenada. At a fabulously posh hotel there called Calabash, he lay on a sunlounger under a tree listening to music. Suddenly there was an almighty crash. A three-foot-long iguana had fallen out of the tree above him, missing his body by inches. It was shocking and hilarious in equal measure, and became a much-repeated holiday story. On my third morning in Negril, I had just settled on a sunbed under a palm tree when two huge, heavy palm fronds fell loudly from the tree above, narrowly missing me. This caused consternation all around. An American man on a nearby bed said, 'That's gotta be a sign of something.' How right he was.

I met up with friends Pamela and Wayne, who we had met there before, played tennis daily, slept and got invitations to join people for dinner. It's my belief that Johnnie looked down and thought, *She's doing just fine*, and allowed himself to go further upward on his journey. And it's true – I had a fantastic holiday and let my hair down for the first time in a year, relieved to no longer have the stress of caring, and also feeling proud that I could still laugh my head off, be it on a tennis court or at the dinner table. It's honestly been quite a revelation to be able to put myself first again.

I've kept myself busy, possibly to avoid the sadness – I don't mind admitting that. However, on three notable occasions I couldn't hold in the emotion. At a church service for the recently bereaved of the Shaftesbury benefice, I started crying as the first hymn began and didn't stop for the entire service. I was on the verge of howling out loud and had to hold it together as much as I could. Then, visiting my mother at her old folk's home in faraway Ludlow, I sat down, having not seen her for almost a year. 'Darling, such a lot has happened since we last saw each other …' I dissolved, realising that the mother–daughter bond, no matter the challenges, remains incredibly deep and profound. And finally, on what would have been Johnnie's eightieth birthday on Sunday, 30 March 2025, his executive producer, Paul Thomas, crafted the most incredible tribute show for Radio 2 (it was Pick of the Day/Week in most papers). That and my own solo tribute show later that evening on Boom Radio was all too much for me in one day – so many amazing memories all packed together. The tears that fell when I went to bed that night were so intense that I simply wished I too was in heaven, holding him. The pain was just too great to bear. I ached because I missed him so much.

Tears remain close to the surface. It's easier when people don't ask about him. I'm learning to put on a tough front. At a recent Radio 2 tribute evening for Steve Wright, where I saw many of Johnnie's old colleagues for the first time since he died, I just used the line, 'Please don't be sorry. His body was at its end. He died just when he should.' And that is the truth. Johnnie was absolutely ready to move on.

A particularly spiritual friend, Clare, has seen Johnnie with Jesus. She was so excited to tell me that he looked ten years younger, he was healthy and handsome, and he told her that he had received the answers to all his questions. I wish I knew what those were. He also told her that he recognised how much I had sacrificed to look after him throughout our marriage, and that now he would devote himself to looking after me. And honestly, I'm taking that. I really have had an inner sense of calm and a belief that it will all be OK, because he is with me.

I speak to him every day. Out loud. And I've started channelling him – not his words, but his behaviour. I'm now regularly late for things, and seem pretty unrepentant. I'm speaking my mind when possibly I shouldn't. I'm forgetting to put things in my diary and double-booking myself as a result. I'm saying 'No' when once I would have said 'Yes'. 'Miss Goody Two-Shoes' is starting to walk on the wild side. I'm not stressing about life as once I did. 'No amount of worrying ever changed tomorrow.' Hallelujah, Duke! Not only am I channelling my inner Johnnie, but I am also receiving the love that was once given to him – from his listeners, the radio world, even some musicians – as if I'm his ambassador or substitute. It's been an unexpected, beautiful bonus. I mean, it's quite something when Bonnie Raitt asks if I'd like to come to her gig in London. The woman behind his 'Oh, Johnnie' jingle. Perhaps it's her recognition that I was the wife she could have been! A DJ and a rock star? It would never have worked …

I've thought quite a lot about fame since Johnnie died. Having a public life is a two-edged sword. It brings some sort of power – to be heard, to be invited, to be read … but it also comes with high stakes, certainly today when the culture is to build people up and then smash them down for the slightest mishap, wrong word or misjudgement. I don't think many people are truly cut out for it. You need to have great innate strength, a toughness and self-belief. Johnnie had that. When he slipped up – and he did – he learned from his mistakes, he repented, and he came back stronger, grateful for a second chance. (I think especially of his cocaine bust, which would have broken most people.) His motivation was never fame or money; it was to share the music that he loved. He came from a pure place. I genuinely believe that his fans and listeners know this. That's why they've been so loyal. They have lost a true friend, just as I've lost a loving husband. This book is for them so they can know him a little better. And honestly, they deserve it in return for the support they have given to both of us. Of course, it has also been cathartic for me. It's kept him with me, reliving our best times together (and a few of the bad).

I look at successful politicians, sportspeople, actors, rock stars, presenters, and I have nothing but admiration for how they cope with their public existence. How frightening and stressful it must sometimes be – especially if they are doing it for the wrong reasons … I loved our final two months together when Johnnie had stepped down from radio. It really was our only 'normal' period. And yet by writing this book I've had to question myself about being a public figure. I'm opening both myself and Johnnie up to criticism and judgement. I hold on to the thought that he was delighted I was writing this. 'Write about whatever you want, Duch. It's your time now.' I thank him still for his belief in me and his love. He knew I was starting to struggle at being the support act for so many years. The narrative was always led by him and his career. Now I'm wholly responsible for what happens next, and there is personal reward in that.

There were so many lasts in 2024. And now, as 2025 unfolds, there are firsts. The first roses, swallows, and … film awards. The short film that I made in the autumn has won me the accolade of Best New Director at the New York Film & Cinematography Awards, the Chicago Indie Film Awards and the Tokyo Indie Shorts Awards. I am quite convinced that Johnnie has had a hand in this from on high. That said, I have stood down as the director of my feature film, *ANTONIA*. Not only am I still too knackered after last year, but the budget level is such that we cannot get the final funding in place with me at the helm. I'm OK with this, but I waited for Johnnie to go before making that decision. I am still the writer and second producer – which will be achievement enough for me.

I cannot deny that it's a relief to have de-medicalised the house – to have the rugs back on the floor; to have a home that is calm, stress-free and tidy. But what I would give to see Johnnie's Lexus come down the drive and him strut his way back into the house wearing jeans and a floral shirt, with a bouquet of flowers in his arms. That's why writing the 'Then' sections of this book has been such a joy, remembering those great days when he could walk and drive, giving me my old Johnnie back. I never realised that basic actions like those were such a privilege.

I will be honest and say that I do not miss the caring. At all. It's tough. To the very end, the only part I truly enjoyed was giving Johnnie a bath. It was intimate and gentle, and he had to be present, not in his bubble. Afterwards he was always grateful because he felt so much better. Yes, bathing someone sick is rewarding.

The house feels big and empty without him – watching television alone in a thirty-three-foot-long room feels a bit echoey – but hopefully it will soon sell, and then I can start again somewhere smaller and cosier. I am sure he has it all planned.

It's a sad process, wrapping up someone's life: to look in a wardrobe once full of fabulous clothes and find only wooden hangers; to close down their phone and email accounts; to feel their existence on this earth slowly evaporate. However, in many ways your relationship continues as you discover new things about them – good and bad! One thing I discovered among his piles of stuff was a cassette tape sat in the top left-hand drawer of his desk. It was labelled 'Duchess 2002'. I'd never seen it before. What a beautiful revelation it was to find this time capsule and hear the songs he had selected for me in those first heady months of our courtship. I am sure he led me to the tape. In what better way could he reveal himself to me than in music?

I loved Johnnie from the moment I met him. Nothing has or ever will change that. I feel immensely lucky to have experienced the one thing in life that we all crave, and to know that it lives on. I believe that one day our souls will be reunited, as they were at the Union Club on 10 September 2001. And when the time comes for me to fall back into his arms, I pray that at our feet will be a little black working cocker spaniel, curving her body, wagging her tail furiously, relieved that our little family is finally back together.

THE HIDDEN 'DUCHESS 2002' CASSETTE

Your final gift to me: a selection of tracks recorded onto a cassette, found three months after you passed – at just the time when I needed you most. Thank you, Duke xx

David Bowie
DRIVE-IN SATURDAY
'Tig the Wonderkid' song.

Hootie & the Blowfish
ONLY WANNA BE WITH YOU
'... you and me, we come from different worlds'.

Stevie Wonder
HE'S MISSTRA KNOW-IT-ALL
Which I dedicated to you on Boom Radio for you were a Mr know-it-all when it came to music.

Van Morrison
BRIGHT SIDE OF THE ROAD

Elton John
YOUR SISTER CAN'T TWIST
(BUT SHE CAN ROCK 'N' ROLL)
A surprising, great-energy choice.

David Bowie and Mick Jagger
DANCING IN THE STREET

The Pretenders
STOP YOUR SOBBING

Paul Simon
THE OBVIOUS CHILD
You always did love a great drum beat.

U2
WHERE THE STREETS HAVE NO NAME

The Who
BABA O'RILEY
Yesssss.

Joe Jackson
STEPPIN' OUT

Bruce Springsteen
BORN TO RUN
Naturally.

Prince
DIAMONDS AND PEARLS
Thank you.

Simon & Garfunkel
KEEP THE CUSTOMER SATISFIED
Great choice.

Christopher Cross
SAILING
Very un-you, but I love it, so thank you.

Rolling Stones
SYMPATHY FOR THE DEVIL

World Party
WAY DOWN NOW
Great to hear again.

Michael Jackson
BLACK OR WHITE
Could have chosen better there, for me.
I'd have preferred 'Earth Song'.

Queen and David Bowie
UNDER PRESSURE
Just a classic.

Simply Red
FAIRGROUND

Eagles
THE LAST RESORT

A perfect end to a fabulous tape – 'call someplace paradise,

kiss it goodbye ...'

TIME PASSAGES – LIFE AFTER JOHNNIE

I stopped turning on the radio at 3 p.m. on a Sunday. I had to. This is no disrespect to Bob Harris who took over Johnnie's BBC *Sounds of the 70s* show, but it was a bit like turning in your bed and seeing the wrong man next to you. Johnnie may have been my husband, but he was also my favourite radio presenter. Yes, he played great music from my top musical decade, but there was something more than that. That voice. He calmed me. His humour was infectious. Even I would hear stories I'd never heard at home. When Johnnie was on air so many people forgot about life for two hours. He was a nationwide panacea, uniting so many of us. Still, over eighteen months since he last broadcast, I feel that something is missing on the radio waves. There's an absence. His unique vibration has gone. I miss that profoundly, and so do many others.

Grief, we are told, is a very individual process. It manifests in different ways and in varying time scales. Looking back, I'd say mine was particularly unusual. I put that down to three reasons. The lead up to his death was intense, stressful and exhausting. I will not be the only full-time carer in the world to think 'thank heavens that ordeal is over' and as an afterthought: 'I'm glad he's no longer suffering.' Johnnie was a public figure so I was very affected by that. He wasn't just a private husband lost. He was a much-mourned national radio legend. There was a lot of other people's grief and emotions to consider. And then there's the fact that I decided to write a book about our life together that was published within nine months of his passing. It was hugely cathartic, and felt like an acknowledgement of both his fans and especially other carers. Yet while I feel justified and indeed proud with my decision to write the book, the process was more all encompassing of my life than I had realised it would be. It didn't leave much space for me to grieve in the traditional sense, or to miss the private man, Duke. It was his public persona that was being grieved.

So, while friends and family looked on with concern and worried about me in my manically busy year, I felt I was keeping Johnnie alive. Every interview I did. Every letter and message I received. Every kind word to me about him as I signed a copy of the book. This was keeping Johnnie as relevant and present as was possible. As such I wasn't really missing him because he was so completely present in my life. Johnnie *was* still my life. Indeed, doing all the radio, press and book tour felt just like our life before, so it was very much my norm – with the one exception – I was the person talking now, not him. Meeting his fans, listening to their stories and hearing their affection for him was wonderful. It was at the Sidmouth Book Festival that a man got to the front of the book signing queue and stood before me in a hugely 'ta da' way. In a split second I knew why. I ran from behind my table and hugged him. He was wearing Johnnie's greatly loved Guillotine blue gilet. He had bought it from me on Vinted! It was like seeing an old friend.

There was just one event in the book process that truly floored me. Reading the audio book. In three days, I sat in a studio in Kilburn with my producer Matt. I was convinced that I would get fired within an hour, not having a drama school training in diction. I was looking for Monica Dolan hidden in the wings. But as it happens she wasn't. My voice passed muster. I was hugely relieved. What I hadn't anticipated was just how overwhelming it would be to read about our twenty-three years together within the space of three days. I broke down time and time again. I couldn't hide my emotion from the microphone. It's true that the mic never lies. You can always hear whether a person is authentic or not. Which is why my editor Katya was so keen that I should narrate it. Matt was a hero. Time and again he said, 'Just take a moment. Have a sip of water. Wipe your eyes …' On day three when I read the section about his death I broke down so much that Matt came into the booth and held me. Truly, we shared such a hugely personal and close three days together that I joked that we should have had a date after that! Strangely, of the entire process, it is the audio book that made me proudest. When I hear from people that they listened for ten hours non-stop without talking, my heart soars.

The year 2025 was also the sixtieth anniversary year of Carers UK, which meant there were even more events than usual to attend throughout the year as Patron of the charity. Again and again, I was digging deep and performing. Reading a particularly brilliant and strong poem about being a carer at their carol service in the Savoy Chapel in December was the one event that almost upended me as the emotion got stuck in my throat. Tears filled my eyes. For a moment I couldn't speak. My friend and actor Pippa Haywood, who was doing another reading, sat in front of me silently willing me on. I got to the end in one piece. Just. But, with the book and the charity, I found that I had plummeted my reserves and cut myself too little time to be still and quiet.

Knowing I would be putting our house on the market, I became a domestically located market trader selling not just Johnnie's stuff that I didn't want to carry into my future, but furniture, books, artwork, etc. I was pragmatic and practical throughout. I was going to buy somewhere smaller and I needed to get rid of the excess. Any meaningful memorabilia I gave to his kids. I just kept his on-stage 'show' outfit, his portrait and his awards. But the truth is that I longed very much to become Tiggy again so that I could be the centre of my own universe.

My big realisation was that while I was still recovering from the fatigue of caring, my tiredness went much further back. Johnnie loved to be contrary. Like the best actors, he had an uncontrollable wildness of spirit. He followed his own path in life no matter what people thought. He would never conform or play the party line. It's one of the characteristics that made him so special, successful and popular. Respected even. He was honest and strong. So not the easiest person to be manager and agent to. Or indeed be married to! Nonetheless, he was without doubt the most profound relationship and teacher in my life. I will always be grateful for that. He opened my eyes and made me more resilient. He taught me just how strong I am. That I can fight and stand up through adversity. Though, honestly, I don't ever want to have to be that strong again.

Feeling I was released from the continual stress of intense caring, meant that I was on some sort of euphoric high for much of the year. You never know there has been a weight on your shoulders until it has been lifted. How I felt that stress fall away. And because he and I both believe the spirit lives on, I did not feel he was gone. Indeed, I spoke to him all the time. He just didn't reply. But then he didn't much when he was here! One of my happiest days was when I got his ashes back. I'd had a terracotta pot made with his name and dates on it, which, until the house sold, sat outside his bedroom window. (He had always said he wanted to be buried under a tree in my garden, but I knew I would be moving so that seemed ill judged.) I asked Dave Holmes the undertaker to come over with *the box*. I know Johnnie lost a lot of weight but there was so little of him in powder form. I poured what there was of him on top of some John Innes No.3 Compost, spread him out with my bare hands, talking to him throughout, added some more compost, and then planted a rose called Rock n Roll on top. Once Dave left I made a cup of tea, took a chair outside and sat with him. 'So, Duke, let me fill you in on what's been going on …' It brought me huge comfort to have him home. I felt safer. More complete. And the rose was happy too.

Anyone who has lost someone they love knows that the year of firsts has to be navigated. This included visiting our old haunts because travelling is really what we did best and when we were at our happiest. Knowing how special our trips to Tresco were, I invited five friends and family to go there so I'd be surrounded by love and jollity in May. Indeed, for two of them, Lisa and Graham, it was their honeymoon. We have always been about the same in tennis, but every day Lisa slaughtered me. By day six I broke down mid-game. I wasn't being a competitive petulant prima donna. It made me realise that I had no fight left in me. And, still, no strength. It was quite shocking for me as I thought I was recovering and on top of things. I know, looking back, that while I felt this huge lifting of stress, I was still suppressing my deepest emotions and my recovery hadn't even started. My fitness and my self-belief were still shattered five months on. It took losing at tennis for me to realise this. However, once the racquets were put away, I supressed that fragility and carried on. There was too much to do to be emotional.

I asked my friends Frank and Rozzi if I could come and stay in Paxos. Another of our special places. There was a certain amount of trepidation from them that I would arrive and mope for three weeks. Far from it. I partied. I laughed. I drank too much. I truly let my hair down. 'Our friend, the grieving widow,' Frank would joke. I was there for 'Irish Week' – when an Irish concert is put on in Loggos. Indeed, I came over with the band on a water taxi from Corfu to Paxos as dusk turned to night. It was beyond special. Paul Brady was the star turn and we talked on the boat about how great Johnnie had been as an interviewer and lover of music. In Paxos I was on some sort of a high. I knew quite a few people there that week, and I discovered just how very kind and generous people are to a new widow. Irish week sparkled. I sparkled. I was so thrilled to be relaxed, happy and free.

There was one evening on Frank and Rozzi's terrace when they had a few friends round for drinks. An evening when I drank on an empty stomach and laughed, joked and was the very life and soul … The next morning, somewhat jaded, Frank shared with me what an astute old university friend had said about me. He told Frank, 'Your friend is coping really well with her loss on the surface. But you can see there's pain underneath.' I was perplexed. I didn't recognise at all that pain he saw. I thought I was fine. Recovered. Just as I'd thought when I'd gone to Tresco – until the tennis games. When the throng of Irish left and I had several days alone on the beach, listening to music tracks that Johnnie and I both loved, the tears then flowed. It was the first time since he had died. Surrounded by couples and families, celebrating the best weeks of their year, I wiped my eyes remembering our happy times together there as I wallowed in Jackson Browne, John Prine, Bonnie Raitt or The Eagles. The astute friend of Frank's appeared to have been right. My euphoria was matched by emotion. (*A warning to men! Don't ever get too close to a woman who has recently been widowed. While she may present as strong and believe that she is, she will deep down be working through so much.*)

Over and again, tears were released by music. In October, Radio 2 put on a tribute show for Johnnie in the Radio Theatre. I had been quite involved, as Paul Thomas, the producer, wanted so desperately for me to be happy with the show. When guitarist Bernard Butler of Suede rehearsed Johnnie's theme tune – Duane Eddy's 'Because They're Young' on his Gretsch hollow body guitar with that 'twang' sound – I immediately had to grab for my tissues. What is it about music that cuts through all the tough front and stiff upper lip I've inherited? Helen Thomas, the Radio 2 controller, immediately sent for Rescue Remedy. Hosted beautifully by Jo Whiley, there were audio tributes from so many great artists. The evening started with an especially touching one from Tim Davey, then Director General. The guests were a mixture of radio folk and musicians. However, the final interview guest was me. I held my own. But more importantly, as the evening came to an end, I felt a line had been drawn. Surely all the remembrance for Johnnie was now done, and I could go forward, privately continuing on my personal quest to mourn my Duke and re-find Tiggy. I was so grateful to Radio 2 for doing this tribute, but I was happy to have reached the end of the public attention.

The real, unrestrained mourning of 'Duke' waited till I collapsed in an exhausted heap in Sydney, eleven and a half months after he passed. I went to spend a month with my brother Graham so that I was away from the UK for the last remaining 'firsts' – our wedding anniversary, Christmas, my birthday and, of course, the anniversary of his death. I cried on all of those remaining firsts. Genuinely. Deeply. Usually alone in my room. But not exclusively. On Christmas evening, sat on Graham's deck with a huge throng of Australian friends and family, sheets of tears slid uncontrollably from my eyes. This emotion was exacerbated by the passing of Graham's wonderful wife Kim who had shockingly died at the start of 2024. Johnnie at the end of it. Everyone individually came and talked to me about the horror of Kim's demise. That somehow helped release me. Together we shared.

I have an extended Australian family based around my brother, my beautiful nieces Brigitte and Georgia, their families, and also Sam, Johnnie's son. Having never referred to him as my 'stepson' I now started to. Days with him out there were so precious. We talked about his father a lot and I let more tears fall. We both benefited from spending time together, not least NYE when I said I wanted to do a post on social media marking the anniversary of his death. Sam elected to be the cameraman instead of being in it. I just sat and spoke. I just let it flow from the heart. Mainly I wanted to express how incredibly moved I was by all the messages of love and support from Johnnie's fans over the year. They had been astonishingly kind, sending me love, checking in to see if I was OK, and leaving wonderful comments about the book. I had never expected that from adversity would come such beauty. I wanted people to know how much I appreciated it. 'Every negative produces a positive' – and this outpouring of love from his fans to me was one of the greatest positives of my year.

I really do consider myself very lucky. I have been held throughout. At the end of my 'queen's speech' when I toasted Johnnie and the New Year, I accidentally knocked my glass of champagne against my leg. Riddled with nervous energy and emotion I laughed out loud. I asked Sam to cut that thinking it undermined what I'd said, but both he and his wife Jules said it should be left in. They were right as that was the bit people liked most – because it was so Johnnie to be laughing at your own mistakes! I've never tried to be a parent to Sam, but I very much wanted to be with him on the anniversary of Johnnie's passing, and going forward to be there even more for him and his family. And since that trip I have been. We are in touch most weeks. Having Sam in my life is one of the best legacies of being married to Johnnie.

With my nieces' children I laughed and played. Who knew Bug Bingo was such fun! It was utterly heart-warming to see bright new lives developing. I don't have kids so I still find it fascinating how early they develop their personalities. Two of the girls, Ella and Florence, learned to surf while I was there. These talented fearless little girls upright on their boards out-doing all the boys. What a proud great aunt I felt. One life goes, others come in. It really is a circle.

There's no doubt that my month in Australia was the punctuation point I needed. I stepped away from my life. Without realising it, I had a deep need to be looked after – and I was by all of them. It was a truly nurturing family trip and started the healing I needed. Without sounding selfish, when you are a carer you do not matter. The focus is almost exclusively on the patient. On this trip it was all about me. I had the solo spotlight and, honestly, that felt good.

On my return in mid-January 2026 I walked straight into a house move. This is something I would not recommend with jetlag. Especially in our winter when the days are wet, cold and dark. The house selling had been a totally stressful nightmare. In November, three days before I was due to complete on the sale of our place, the chain of six houses tripped up due to the buyer at the bottom of the chain. Because I am a hopeless optimist, and because I was going away to Australia for five weeks, I went ahead with the move out and into storage, as I was certain it was just a temporary blip. Happily, I wasn't buying my next house until early January, but because I knew that house was my destiny, I had thrown the dice and agreed to exchange on the day of my supposed completion, come what may. Before flying off

I temporarily moved in with brother Martin and his wife Kate. They looked after me like a broken bird. Martin cooked amazing meals and Kate would do my laundry and clean my bathroom. I did joke that I might stay. And a bit of me meant it. Having been alone for eleven months it was fabulous to have company again, to share, and to have balanced conversations with equals about non-health-related matters.

I returned time and again to the empty house to check all was OK. On every occasion I thanked the building for keeping us so safe and protecting Johnnie. And every day away in Australia I hoped for good news. It never came. And then, almost two months later than the original completion date, in which time I had taken an almighty loan combined with many prayers, I finally said goodbye to the house for the final time. As I drove away from it and all the memories it held, from kitchen discos to death, I real-ised something extraordinary – it was exactly one year after his funeral to the day. That JW timing again.

The house I have bought is the most perfect fit for me, the self-confessed house snob. It is the greatest possible way to restart my life. It is rural, hidden, stunningly designed, renovated to the highest standard and utterly charming. Made of cream Chilmark stone, it is T-shaped with a wide front door under a porch, with a slate roof and pretty dormer windows upstairs. It would certainly give the cottage used in *The Holiday* a run for its money. Incredibly, Johnnie saw it in the days when he could still walk. We'd offered on it a few years before but our sale then hadn't worked out. I remember the day we went to see it. As we drove up the drive my jaw dropped. I told him, 'We don't need to go in. I can already tell you that I want to live here.' It was even lovelier inside. 'I could sit here and look at that view for the rest of my life,' I uttered as I gazed across a far-reaching green valley edged with deciduous woods. The house was rented out instead of being sold. In his last couple of months Johnnie said, in his customary financially cavalier fashion, 'I know it's more than you should spend on a house, but you love it. Go and get it Duch. You'd be so happy there.' And, as if by fate, I did go and get it. It had waited for me.

When people visit and tell me how lucky I am, I wholeheartedly agree. I also say – I've earned this. A further joy is that now all my possessions are under one roof, having also sold our London flat in among the frantic year. It made me stupidly happy to unwrap the wine and champagne glasses from London that we bought when we first married in 2002. I can only assume they survived as we often ate out when in town. This darling house represents the sum of my life and who I am. Every painting, rug, piece of furniture – and glass. It's like a completed jigsaw. Indeed, it is so me that it feels as if the previous owners renovated it specifically for me. This is fate. The biggest symbol that my life ahead is going to be good. I am safe. This house is healing me.

What is more, there's still plenty to smile about with Johnnie – and his shopping addiction. Granted, I was combining two homes but still … seventeen torches, fourteen walking sticks (he never went for walks!), thirteen pairs of scissors, enough leads and cables to run IBM, so many tools like screwdrivers and sets of heads that I could open a hardware shop, bulbs of every type, boxes and boxes of face masks (he never wore one!) and heat patches, two rammed-full drawers of pens and highlighters, nine staplers, multiple tubes of Berocca … There are many things I will never ever have to purchase again. Thank you, Johnnie.

One way I have changed is that having vowed to him that I never wanted another relationship, even though he said I should, I have now decided it might be OK. Fun even. Not in the full-blown marriage/living together way. (I'm enjoying now being single and selfish too much.) But a smattering of romance wouldn't go amiss. All the time I was with Johnnie I was utterly loyal. My head was never turned. Now I know it could be.

I have frequently questioned why Johnnie and I came together having been such strong opposites. Then, more than a year after he passed, I was delivered a realisation when I spoke to Jean the Medium. Of the many things she told me, one thing truly struck a chord. In this life I was repaying a karmic debt to Johnnie. He had saved my life in a previous existence, and in this one it was my turn to save him. Everything fell into place. There is no doubt that some people possess psychic powers. I include in that my healer Alice in Wilton. I have seen her five times in the past year. At every occasion Johnnie has been present. The first time she said he was in the room with us. The following times he was further and further away, sometimes just coming in to acknowledge us. But shortly after I had returned from Australia and got through the appalling stress of selling our house, our flat and moving into my new one; having survived financially by the skin of my teeth, Alice heard him speak as clear as a bell, with his wonderful voice as if he were in the room. He said, '*Tiggy, I am so proud of you.*'

Perhaps he hadn't realised my strength before now. It made me think of the time years ago when he popped into Elstree Studios where I was producing a TV commercial for Carphone Warehouse. It was a huge set, and there were over eighty crew working on it. He asked, 'Are you in charge of all this?' I said that I was – being the producer. He took my hands and looked down into my eyes and said incredulously, 'But you're so small!' Johnnie came from a time when most men considered themselves more capable than women. I am from a time when we know that not to be the case. Since his death I have pulled through every challenge and kept smiling. He has looked down at this, and I know he has been impressed. So, of all the things that have been said to me by anyone since he died, those seven words from him '*Tiggy, I am so proud of you*' mean more to me than anything.

And I am still proud of him. When Neil Sedaka died, on BBC Sounds, Radio 2 re-ran an in-depth interview Johnnie had done with him. It was an exquisite pleasure for me to hear him doing what he did best when he was at the top of his game. It was quite simply a masterclass in how to do a musical interview.

As for my future … I have complete faith. I have reached a place of total acceptance. If things are supposed to happen – they will. If my film *ANTONIA* is supposed to happen, it will. If I am supposed to write another book, I will (I've a novel in me screaming to be written). If I'm supposed to do some more radio, I will. If I am supposed to experience love again, I will. I can now listen to Radio 2 at 3 p.m. on a Sunday. Fear has left me. Stress has left me. I survived an enormous and challenging chapter with darling Johnnie. If I could survive that, I can survive anything. I wish I could share with you this feeling of calm optimism combined with how loved I feel. It is such an overwhelmingly real sensation that I can honestly say – I have never been happier. Maybe that's why he's so proud of me.

THANK YOUS

This book would never have been born had it not been for my dear old friend from Bristol University days, the incredibly talented and successful novelist Rachel Joyce. Despite her great stature in literary circles, she has always believed in me and my writing. She contacted me in June 2024, the day after I had been on the Jeremy Vine Radio 2 show, and in the middle of the terrible caring year. 'Are you writing about this time?' she asked. I told her I was not. 'Should I?' 'Yes,' she said firmly. 'I believe you have something to say that hasn't been said before and I know you will do so with the right touch.' High praise indeed. I started writing that night.

Carly Cook has been a friend since she edited Johnnie's autobiography in 2007. She and I went through breast cancer together and she has been down to stay with us several times since. She contacted me after I had been on Times Radio with Fi Glover – about a month after the Jeremy Vine show. She loved that I'd mentioned Johnnie having a crafty fag outside – with lung disease! 'I don't suppose you're writing about this time?' Thanks to Rachel,

I was. She asked to be my agent on the spot. Some things are meant to be. Carly has been such a support, not just with the book and securing HarperCollins as the right publishing house for this, but also emotionally. She's incredibly protective. An attack dog who kept the paps at the funeral at a respectful distance, and a passionate fighter who is incredible to have just over your shoulder.

Thank you to Katya Shipster, my editor, who has shown me why everyone always thanks their editor. It has been like the most intense therapy session, and I am indebted to her for her astute questions and fabulous guidance, not least cutting out the parts that were 'TMI' – too much information. All her notes were amazing – the good and the bad ones. To Daisy Ward and Holly Kyte for all their editing and checks – especially spelling! And to the HarperCollins marketing team – Alex Layt and Chris Kwok, who have helped spread the word.

To the island of Tresco, in particular Dean Whillis, who gave me a refuge to run to after the funeral and write. It was the most perfect place to re-find my equilibrium and tap away. I will always be grateful to all the islanders who embraced and supported me – notably Anna Parkes, my dear friend who runs Tresco Gallery in the finest array of clothes ever seen. She is an inspiration. Her story is even more interesting than ours!

To my dear, mainly local, girlfriends who have kept me afloat during the caring year and since – Jane Treays, Susan d'Arcy, Jacquie Glanville, Camilla Royce, Sarah Tanner,

Lesley Waters, Lisa Linde, Clare Galtrey and all the fabulous tennis gang. You have kept me sane and loved. Thank you so much. Many of you helped look after Johnnie when I had moments of respite, along with my brother Martin Coldicott and his wife, Kate, Sophie Bainsfair, Claire Hooper, Margaret Millward, Lisa Supple, Virginia Edwyn-Jones, Rodney Wayman, Tommy and Mairead King, Tim McPherson, Beth and Mariana. You gave me much-needed freedom to grab gulps of air. You never questioned giving support and fed Johnnie bloody well!

A thank you to Johnnie's listeners and fans for your love and support. You know who you are. And the thousands of you who send us/me cards, letters and messages on social media – it's like we are friends. I feel blessed to have your strength behind me. I wrote this book for you – so I hope you enjoyed it.

To all who have given me spiritual and emotional healing: Alice Young, Sarah Lownds, Richard Sutton and shaman Anna Hunt.

To Liz 'Queen of Rock' Barnes, Johnnie's producer, for being so patient with his illness, and for reminding me who played at the Peter Green Tribute Show so I could make myself sound like a Princess of Rock in the 'Stardust' chapter. And to executive producer Paul Thomas for knowing that you should be there for the final show, making the amazing tribute shows and keeping a gentle eye on me since. I hope we work together again. You are full of great ideas, music knowledge and compassion.

To Helen Thomas and Radio 2 for the love and support before and after. You have all made me feel like a part of the Radio 2 family. And not just a distant aunt. I have really felt embraced by you all and your love of dear Johnnie.

Mark and Jacqueline Goodier. Oh, you two. So kind, so supportive, so there for us both. Always. Your calmness in our lives has been such a blessing.

To Frank and Rozzi Musker for embracing me into their beautiful Paxos life to recover.

To Johnnie's son Sam, his nieces Trudi and Michelle, and his cousin Mal – thank you for your love and care during and since.

Most of all I have to thank my subject: Johnnie – my Duke – Walker. Without you, darling, I'd have no book. By writing it, I have felt almost as close to you as when you were here. How wonderful to relive our adventure. You gave me one hell of a ride.